ON THE FOUNDATIONAL PRINCIPLES OF REHABILITATION PSYCHOLOGY

ACADEMY OF REHABILITATION PSYCHOLOGY SERIES

Series Editors

Volumes in the Series

Ethics Field Guide: Applications in Rehabilitation Psychology
Thomas R. Kerkhoff and Stephanie L. Hanson

The Social Psychology of Disability
Dana S. Dunn

Disability-Affirmative Therapy: A Case Formulation Template for Clients with Disabilities
Rhoda Olkin

Validity Assessment in Rehabilitation Psychology and Settings
Dominic A. Carone and Shane S. Bush

Suicide Prevention after Neurodisability: An Evidence-Informed Approach
Grahame K. Simpson and Lisa A. Brenner

Understanding the Experience of Disability: Perspectives from Social and Rehabilitation Psychology
Dana S. Dunn

Disability as Diversity: Developing Cultural Competence
Erin E. Andrews

Teaching Disability: Practical Activities for In Class and Homework
Rhoda Olkin

Critical Care Psychology and Rehabilitation: Principles and Practice
Kirk J. Stucky and Jennifer E. Jutte

Motivational Interviewing in Medical Rehabilitation: Improving Patient Engagement and Team Function
Nicole Schechter, Connie Jacocks, Lester Butt, and Stephen T. Wegener

On the Foundational Principles of Rehabilitation Psychology: Origins, Understanding, and Applications
Dana S. Dunn

On the Foundational Principles of Rehabilitation Psychology

ORIGINS, UNDERSTANDING, AND APPLICATIONS

Dana S. Dunn

OXFORD
UNIVERSITY PRESS

OXFORD
UNIVERSITY PRESS

Oxford University Press is a department of the University of Oxford. It furthers the University's objective of excellence in research, scholarship, and education by publishing worldwide. Oxford is a registered trade mark of Oxford University Press in the UK and in certain other countries.

Published in the United States of America by Oxford University Press
198 Madison Avenue, New York, NY 10016, United States of America.

CIP data is on file at the Library of Congress.

ISBN 9780197785157

DOI: 10.1093/9780197785188.001.0001

Printed by Marquis Book Printing, Canada

The manufacturer's authorized representative in the EU for product safety is
Oxford University Press España S.A., Parque Empresarial San Fernando de Henares,
Avenida de Castilla, 2 – 28830 Madrid (www.oup.es/en or product.safety@oup.com).
OUP España S.A. also acts as importer into Spain of products made by the manufacturer.

MIX
Paper | Supporting responsible forestry
FSC www.fsc.org FSC® C103567

In memory of my friend, John Patrick Crecine,
who saw possibilities in me that I did not.

Contents

Foreword by Lisa A. Brenner, Ph.D

PERHAPS NOW, MORE than at any time in the recent past, it is vital that we as clinicians, scientists, educators, and policy makers use history as a guiding light. In his newest contribution to the Oxford University Press Rehabilitation Psychology Series, titled *On the Foundational Principles of Rehabilitation Psychology: Origins, Understanding, and Applications*, Dr. Dunn provides the reader with both vital information regarding the foundational principles of rehabilitation psychology and guidance in regard to how these can be used to increase cultural competence about the "nature, meaning, experience, and understanding of disability and chronic health issues" and be applied in everyday practice. Dr. Dunn starts by setting the historical stage (Chapter 1), introducing the reader to the early ideas in the field (precursors to the foundational principles). Chapters that follow provide sophisticated, yet accessible, discussions on key topics (e.g., "Disability as Diversity" [Chapter 2], "Self-Perception of Bodily States" [Chapter 7], and "The Importance of Human Dignity" [Chapter 8]). Then, before integrating the information presented throughout to help professionals leverage foundational principles in everyday practice (e.g., education/training; "The Primacy of the Foundational Principles," Chapter 10]), Dr. Dunn reminds us about the importance of "Advocacy: Now and Always" (Chapter 9). In reading this chapter, I connected with my own professional origins. *Why rehabilitation psychology?* Growing up, the concept of *tikkun olam*, which literally means "world repair" but has become synonymous with social action and social justice, played a pivotal role in shaping my development. Highlighting both priorities for disability advocacy and justice, Dr. Dunn's words provide direction and clarity, as well as inspiration. Reading Dr. Dunn's words, I was once again reminded that advocacy is a key component of my work as a rehabilitation psychologist. I hope other readers will feel the same and, in doing so, use information regarding our shared history and foundational principles to advocate for a present and future in which all people are treated with respect and dignity.

Lisa A. Brenner, Ph.D
Professor of Physical Medicine and Rehabilitation
University of Colorado Anschutz Medical Campus
Aurora, Colorado

Preface and Acknowledgments

GUSTAV FLAUBERT— who was not a psychologist but often thought like one—wrote, "The art of writing is the art of discovering what you believe." What could be truer than that?

My belief in writing about and sharing psychological science to understand the experience of disability and to promote the practice and science of rehabilitation psychology is stronger than ever. The field of rehabilitation psychology tacitly codified a group of foundational principles that are grounded in clinical, practice, research, and advocacy efforts as well as the social psychology of disability. These principles are drawn from the work of the social psychologist Kurt Lewin and his students Beatrice A. Wright, Roger G. Barker, and Tamara Dembo, among others, who founded and shaped this essential subfield of American psychology.

The principles can help disabled persons develop a positive disability identity while also promoting or maintaining resilience when encountering obstacles and challenges linked to disability. For their part, nondisabled people can reduce their ableist beliefs and become disability allies by learning about the foundational principles. Elucidating and reflecting on the foundational principles allowed me to better appreciate their breadth, scope, and genuine applicability and to improve my understanding of the experience of disability from both biopsychosocial and intersectional perspectives. The foundational principles also present the opportunity for interested individuals to become more culturally competent about the nature, meaning, experience, and understanding of disability and chronic health issues.

The primary audiences for *On the Foundational Principles* are research psychologists, clinicians, educators, and graduate students in rehabilitation psychology and researchers and graduate students in disability studies, social psychology, and health psychology, as well as aligned fields (e.g., social work, nursing, rehabilitation sciences). Policy makers and undergraduate students in psychology or related fields may also be interested. Disabled people themselves, their families and caregivers, and casual readers might also want to learn about the importance and applicability of the foundational principles toward improving living with disability. Any errors or omissions in the book are, of course, mine.

The genesis of this book came about through my earlier research, writing, and speaking, as well as my participation in Division 22 (Rehabilitation Psychology) of the American Psychological Association and my service on the board of the Foundation for Rehabilitation Psychology. I continue to appreciate and benefit from the professional fellowship offered by these groups and their members. I also want to thank a particular circle of friends for their enthusiasm and critical perspectives on the principles, rehabilitation matters, and disability issues generally, including Daniel Rohe, Timothy Elliott, Bruce Caplan, Lisa Brenner, Dawn Ehde, Stephen Wegener, Katheleen Bogart, Gitendra Uswatte, Barry Nierenberg, Allen Heinemann, Michelle Fine, Bob Frank, John Corrigan, Erin Andrews, Susan Opotow, Joseph Rath, Catherine Wilson, Kate Brown, Michelle Nario-Redmond, Michael Wehmeyer, Kara Ayers, Jan Tackett, Scott Richards, Terrie Price, Susanne Bruyere, Michele Rusin, Mary Brownsberger, Christine Abraham, Carrie Pilarski, Linda Mona, and Anjali Forber-Pratt. I am still learning from them all and am grateful for the opportunity to do so.

I thank Moravian University, especially the members of the Tenure, Promotion, and Review Committee, as well as my department colleagues, for granting me a sabbatical leave for the spring semester of 2024. I wrote this book during that time and through the summer months of 2024. Many friends and colleagues at Moravian support my scholarly efforts, especially Carol Traupman-Carr, Claudia Mesa, Sonia Aziz, Bryon Grigsby, Deb Wetcher-Hendricks, Susan Scholtz, and Stacey Zaremba. I also want to acknowledge former colleagues Michelle Schmidt, Cynthia Kosso, and the late Gordy Weil.

I offer special thanks to Lisa Brenner, who encouraged me to write the book as part of the Academy of Rehabilitation Psychology's series with Oxford University Press

(OUP). At OUP, I appreciate my editor, Nadina Persaud, for her confidence in this as well as my other writing projects, and the professional efforts of Phoebe Aldridge-Turner. I am grateful to Gangaa Radjacoumar of Integra for handling the book's production and to Ruth Saavedra for her skilled copyediting of the manuscript.

My family—Jacob, Stefana, Annaliese, and Lucas Dunn and Hannah, Esteban, and Lilah Angeles—cheered on my efforts, as did my dog, Arno. My dear friend, David Raves, stepped in and up while I recovered from hip surgery in January 2024, just after the book project was underway.

I am a bit tardy in thanking the late Pat Crecine for his kindness and encouragement all those long years ago—here, at last, a dedication to mark his dedication. My heart really is in the work, which I hope will be of help and of use to others.

Dana S. Dunn, Ph.D
Bethlehem, Pennsylvania

There is an old Greek saying that men are tormented not by things themselves but by what they think about them.

Michel de Montaigne (1580)

1 Setting the Stage

PRECURSORS TO THE FOUNDATIONAL PRINCIPLES

Rehabilitation Psychology and the Foundational Principles

Alexis Kashar, a civil rights lawyer, entrepreneur, and member of the Deaf community, was quoted in the *New York Times* (2024) regarding a novel intervention designed to potentially eliminate deafness in some people:

> I question the ethics of the new experimental gene therapy treatment for deafness. The Deaf community has a painful history of being experimented on, often without our consent. Being a native signer of one of the world's most beautiful languages—American Sign Language—I have access to a life that no spoken language can replicate, and I embrace everything about my identity.

This quote illustrates a powerful perspective that is challenging for many people to accept: Some disabled persons do not want to have their disability altered through medical or technological intervention. In other words, deafness—or any other disability for that matter—is a source of positive identity (and here so is American Sign Language [ASL]), a quality that ties individuals together by acknowledging their commonalities. Kashar expresses both pride in and solidarity with other Deaf persons, finding joy in using a particular visual and dynamic form of communication.

On the Foundational Principles of Rehabilitation Psychology. Dana S. Dunn, Oxford University Press.
 DOI: 10.1093/9780197785188.003.0001

Unfortunately, many nondisabled people assume that people with disabilities would prefer to be "cured" or to somehow have their disabilities medically changed or even repaired. To be fair, the disabled community fills a big tent, both in the United States and globally, as it were, and points of view are diverse, not homogeneous. This book is about a set of guiding—that is, foundational—principles that were designed to promote disability as a positive mode of life, one that, as we will learn, nonetheless prompts a variety of pertinent questions.

How should people with disabilities navigate their physical, social, and psychological worlds? How should they think about themselves and their place in the spheres of work, family, friends, and their communities? How, too, should they expect to be treated by the nondisabled people they encounter, including medical and rehabilitation professionals?

In turn, how should nondisabled people learn to understand and affirm disability as a quality like any other that some of their fellow citizens possess? How can nondisabled persons recognize disability as another way of being rather than a source of curiosity or, worse, negativity and even prejudice and discrimination? These and related questions have been asked repeatedly by many disabled individuals, rehabilitation psychologists, and other professionals who work with and for disabled persons, as counselors, practitioners, researchers, colleagues, friends, and allies.

To constructively address these and related questions and concerns, the field of rehabilitation psychology (see, for example, Brenner et al., 2019; Elliott & Rath, 2012; Meade et al., in press) has codified a group of foundational principles that are grounded in clinical and practice efforts as well as the social psychology of disability (Andrews et al., 2023; Dunn et al., 2016). Rehabilitation psychology is focused on the examination and application of psychological data and skills to benefit people with disabilities and chronic health issues to promote their health and well-being, choices and independence, functional capacities, and social connections across the lifespan (Division 22, 2024). The principles were drawn from the work of the social psychologist Kurt Lewin, and some of his students, including Beatrice A. Wright, Tamara Dembo, and Roger Barker, who helped to found and shape the field of rehabilitation psychology. The related efforts of these and other psychologists who shaped the theory and practice of rehabilitation psychology will also be considered in this book (e.g., Trieschmann, 1988; Vash, 1981; Vash & Crewe, 2004). Indeed, as Roger Barker (1960, p. xiii) wrote,

> Human physique has a central place in naïve, commonsense psychology. It is generally believed that a person's body influences his behavior by way of the many phenomenal properties it has for him and his associates, and by way

of it greater or lesser efficiency as the instrument with which he attempts to carry out intended actions.

To begin, we should define what we mean by disability before turning to how the principles came into being.

Disability Defined

Disabilities come in various forms; they can be physical, sensory, and intellectual, and some are invisible (i.e., not apparent to observers, or "hidden"), psychiatric, or due to a chronic health condition, among other possibilities. Disabilities can be broadly understood as being of two types: congenital or acquired. A congenital disability is a quality that a person has had since birth (e.g., deafness), while an acquired disability is one that occurs at some point in the person's life (e.g., limb loss due to an industrial accident in the workplace). In both cases, the term "disability" is linked to a particular person and, as a result, is to some degree embodied—that is, personified—by the individual. Disabilities exist when routine activities people do are limited or somehow constrained (e.g., speaking, walking, reading, watching) so that they cannot be done in an accustomed or familiar manner.

Terms like "impairment" and "handicap" are often used as interchangeable synonyms for "disability" in everyday language (Livneh & Antonak, 1997), but they do not share the same meaning. "Impairment" is a technical term (found in the International Classification of Function) that refers to disruption at the system level of an organ in the body (e.g., the brain, an arm, a leg) leading to a loss or a detected abnormality (i.e., a deviation from some established norm but by no means a "defect") whose nature is tied to anatomy, physiology, or psychology (World Health Organization, 2001). Generally, impairments tend to be lasting states, if not always permanent ones, that occur following the onset of disease or an injury. Impairments are consequential, however, as they disrupt the affected person's physical, cognitive, and/or emotional processes (Livneh, 1987).

What about the term "handicap?" This term highlights the presence of some obstacle in the environment that affects some people by preventing them from completing desired goals or filling a particular role (World Health Organization, 2001). Use of the word "environment" is important, as it can point to challenging terrain or some situational constraint, such as a literal structural feature or one that is missing. Older structures, including historic ones, that have never been retrofitted often create accessibility and egress barriers for wheelchair users, for example, as does curbing in public places that lack curb cuts. Under such circumstances, a wheelchair user is *handicapped* by the absence of an elevator, a ramp, or similar. Please note that the person using the wheelchair is not handicapped per se; rather, the handicapping aspect is present in the environment confronting the person but not in the person themselves. Most built environments were designed for nondisabled persons, not disabled ones; had the environment in question been an accommodating one, the individual would not have been handicapped by it. As a social and rehabilitation psychologist, Beatrice A. Wright (1983) acknowledged that environmental handicaps also can be interpersonal in nature, as in the case of devaluing or negative attitudes held by nondisabled others, which can affect social life, education, economic advancement, and emotional support.

THE WHO ICF MODEL

Distinguishing meaning among terms like "disability," "impairment," and "handicap," as well as acknowledging the importance of the environment (actual as well as perceived, physical as well as social and psychological), is relevant for understanding the WHO International Classification of Functioning, Disability, and Heath (ICF) model (World Health Organization, 2001; see also Dunn, 2015, 2019a). This model provides a universal classification system that can be applied to all levels of health and well-being, not exclusively disability or chronic illness. The model is biopsychosocial by design, which means that disabilities or chronic illnesses are not based exclusively on biological processes. To properly understand the experience of people with disabilities, attention must focus on the interactions among biological, psychological, and social systems factors (e.g., Rath & Elliott, 2011; Rath et al., in press).

The overarching goal of the ICF model and classification is to expand theory, research, practice efforts, and policy initiatives to enhance the lives of people with disabilities, thereby ensuring that they are very much a part of mainstream society (Bruyère & Peterson, 2005; Peterson & Rosenthal, 2005). The model construes disability as falling on a continuum where each affected individual reacts and functions in a unique way because of the interaction between personal and environmental factors (see Figure 1.1). As contextual influences, both *environmental factors* (e.g., physical or structural, attitudinal, familial, cultural, social, institutional, technological) and *personal factors* (e.g., gender, personality, age, education, profession, lifestyle, additional health-related qualities, coping style, reactions to stressors) are key because they can change or affect the model's other components. In fact, the term "disability" is characterized as "the outcome or result of a complex relationship between an individual's health condition and personal factors, and of the external factors that represent the circumstances in which the individual lives"

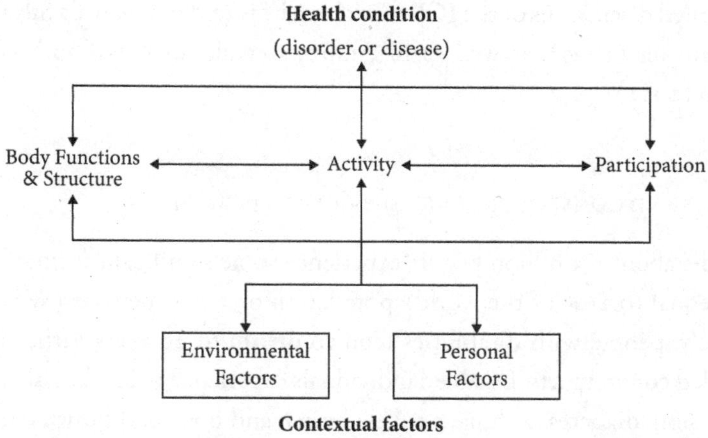

FIGURE 1.1 The WHO ICF Model of Disability

(World Health Organization, 2001, p. 17). As we will learn, this definition fits with the Lewinian perspective in social psychology and rehabilitation psychology known as the *person-environment relation*, one of the foundational principles (which will be introduced briefly below and discussed in detail in Chapter 3; see also Lewin, 1935).

As Figure 1.1 illustrates, the experience of disability is dynamic, potentially involving interactions between *health conditions* (e.g., disorders, diseases, injuries) and the aforementioned *contextual factors* tied to the person and the environment. A person's health condition or impairment and contextual factors can influence body functions and structure, activity, and participation. Body functions entail both psychological and physiological functions of systems within the body. *Body structures* refer to anatomical parts of the body, such as limbs, organs, and components within each. Both functions and structures represent the system levels in which impairment can take place. *Activity* encompasses the way a person performs an action or finishes some behavioral tasks. Someone experiencing *activity limitations* can face challenges executing actions or completing a task due to a disability. *Participation* acknowledges the person's involvement in some life situation where activities take place (e.g., shopping, preparing a meal, studying for an exam, exercising, socializing). Disabled individuals sometimes experience problems in some life situations when an environmental constraint causes *participation restriction*, a referent designed to replace the more familiar, if dated and pejorative, term "handicap" (recall the discussion above). Yet the model posits, for example, that a disabled person may have significant impairment while still presenting qualities tied to favorable health and well-being (Andrews et al., in press). Disability can occur in any of the levels of the ICF model (i.e., impairments, activity limitations, and/or participation restrictions).

More detailed discussions of the ICF model can be found in Chan, da Silva Cordoso, and Chronister (2009), as well as in Andrews et al. (in press) and Wehmeyer and Dunn (2022).

INCIDENCE AND CONSEQUENCES OF DISABILITY: IN BRIEF

Worldwide, about 1.3 billion people experience some significant form of disability, which is equal to 16% of the world's population or 1 in 6 persons (WHO, 2023). Collectively, people with disabilities tend to die up to 20 years earlier than their nondisabled counterparts. Disabled individuals experience twice the risk of developing depression, diabetes, asthma, stroke, obesity, and poor oral health compared to nondisabled people. Not surprisingly, perhaps, people with disabilities face serious and unfair health inequities that are fueled by social stigma, discrimination, barriers to education and employment, poverty, and deficiencies in available health care systems (WHO, 2023).

Disability, then, is clearly a global health concern. Bentley and colleagues (2019) outlined a variety of disability-related healthcare needs. In the first place, civil societies should work to improve the inclusion of people with disabilities, especially when it comes to making services available to enhance their health and well-being in daily life. Too often, disabled people's circumstances are evaluated exclusively in medical terms (e.g., as a health problem), or their abilities to navigate everyday life are seen as less competent than those of nondisabled persons (e.g., Dunn, 2019b,c). Around the world, available public services for disabled persons vary greatly due to culture, country, and custom; they are often inadequate or unavailable (WHO, 2013).

As Bentley and colleagues (2019) noted, too, poverty and employment equity are also serious concerns linked to disability. Globally, disabled individuals are at greater risk for living in impoverished circumstances than are nondisabled people. Influential factors leading to this outcome include limited access to education, fewer opportunities to develop needed skills, and a lack of available or productive employment prospects. When employment is secured, people with disabilities often experience discrimination in hiring, as well as underemployment, low compensation, limitations to career growth, and gender inequity (i.e., disabled women struggle more to find decent jobs than nondisabled individuals; see Lindstrom et al., 2013). Not surprisingly, there are social as well as psychological consequences for such discriminatory treatment. Due to being marginalized or overlooked, some disabled people lose confidence and settle for less-than-ideal employment, if any, instead of venturing outside their familiar settings.

What about disabled people who live in the United States? Much of what we have just covered holds true for disabled Americans. Approximately 13.5% of US citizens have some form of disability, and 46% of those who are aged 75 years or over live with a disability (Statista, 2024). However, the United States has had decades of social activism aimed at improving the lives of disabled citizens. The Americans with Disabilities Act, which became law in July 1990, has helped to improve the lives of those who live with disability, especially where presence and inclusion are concerned (e.g., National Council on Disability, 2007). At the same time, problems including employment discrimination and hiring challenges, especially where individuals with visible or severe disabilities are concerned, remain. Educational opportunity and economic self-sufficiency remain tenuous for many disabled Americans (e.g., Dunn, 2015). For more detail on the epidemiology of disability and health issues, see Dixon-Ibarra et al., 2019; for assessment of and intervention for disability, see Hanson et al., 2023.

The need to identify and articulate values or principles to constructively guide disabled people and their nondisabled allies is important. We turn now to the history of what have become known as the foundational principles in rehabilitation psychology.

Origins of the Foundational Principles

In 1972, Beatrice A. Wright wrote an article that outlined what she then referred to as "value-laden beliefs and principles for rehabilitation psychology." These beliefs and principles were created to affirm the human and civil rights of disabled people, helping them to speak out and to engage in acts of self-determination for themselves. Wright identified 18 guiding principles that expanded a list of 12 from an earlier publication (see Wright, 1959). Later, in 1980, Shontz and Wright revised and updated the beliefs and principles. Shortly thereafter, Wright (1983) published the second edition of her seminal book, *Physical Disability: A Psychosocial Approach*, which expanded them to 20 and presented them in the work's preface. Importantly, the last entry in the list stated, "*Continuing review of the contributions of psychologists and others in rehabilitation within a framework of guiding principles that are themselves subject to review is an essential part of the self-correcting effort of science and the professions*" (Wright, 1983, p. xvii, italics in original).

By then, Wright strongly believed that the problems posed by disability should be clearly understood by the way people—disabled or not—interacted with their real and perceived social environments. She wanted the continually cultivated list of value-laden beliefs and principles to represent constructive views of how to live with disability. To that end, on page xi of the preface, Wright wrote of the value-laden beliefs and principles that

> they are offered as possible guidelines with the intent that they be examined and improved, then kept in the forefront to remind and to prompt, to check and to challenge, lest they remain inactivated and submerged by the weight of social, political, and personal pressures of all sorts.

That ongoing process of reflection and revision continued (see also Wright, 1987)—and continues—which leads us to the current set of guiding principles.

THE CURRENT PRINCIPLES

The current formulation of the foundational principles, which are listed and defined in Table 1.1, include (a) the person-environment relation, (b) the insider-outsider distinction, (c) adjustment to disability, (d) psychological assets, (e) self-perception of bodily states, and (f) human dignity (see Bentley et al., 2019; Dunn et al., 2016; Dunn et al., 2021). Advocacy, including self-advocacy by people with disabilities and that conducted by allies, is also considered to be a seventh additional and important principle (see Table 1.1; Andrews et al., 2023; Dunn et al., 2021). To be sure, this is a smaller subset of principles than the one that Wright (1983) last provided.

The aim of such brevity is to make the principles readily accessible, practical, and useful to new generations of disabled persons, their families, and allies and to help rehabilitation practitioners and researchers (and social, personality, and health psychologists), as well as other interested professionals (e.g., medicine, nursing, social work, health care policy, human resources) provide key services. The current principles can help disabled persons develop a positive disability identity or self-image while also promoting or maintaining resilience when encountering obstacles and challenges linked to disability. Nondisabled people, too, should have a stake in better understanding and appreciating disability as way of being and a form of diversity like many others (see Chapter 2). By doing so, many forms of misunderstanding, not to mention prejudice and discrimination, could be reduced. And, in any case, earlier iterations of the value-laden beliefs and principles remain available to add supporting commentary and detail for the contemporary list shown in Table 1.1.

To advance these ends, each principle has a dedicated chapter in this book where its contributions and constructive implications will be discussed. As a starting point

TABLE 1.1

The Foundational Principles of Rehabilitation Psychology

Principle	Definition
1. Person-environment relation	Attributions about people with disabilities tend to focus on presumed dispositional rather than available situational characteristics. Environmental constraints usually matter more than personality factors to living with a disability.
2. Insider-outsider distinction	People with disabilities (*insiders*) know what life with a chronic condition is like (e.g., sometimes challenging but usually manageable), whereas casual observers (*outsiders*) who lack relevant experience presume that disability is defining, all-encompassing, and decidedly negative.
3. Adjustment to disability	Coping with a disability or chronic illness is an ongoing dynamic process, one dependent on making constructive changes to the social and physical environment.
4. Psychological assets	People with disabilities possess or can acquire personal or psychological qualities that can ameliorate challenges posed by disability and also enrich daily living.
5. Self-perception of bodily states	Experience of bodily states (e.g., pain, fatigue, distress) is based on people's perceptions of the phenomena, not exclusively on the actual sensations. Changing attitudes, expectations, or environmental conditions can constructively alter perceptions.
6. Human dignity	Regardless of the source or severity of a disability or chronic health condition, all people deserve respect and encouragement and to be treated with dignity.
7. Advocacy efforts	Advocacy efforts aimed at promoting the health and well-being of disabled individuals are important. Such efforts should be made by disabled people themselves as well as their allies (e.g., family, friends, medical and rehabilitation professionals).

Note: Adapted from Andrews, Pilarski, Ayers, & Dunn (2023); Dunn et al. (2016).

now, however, the principles can be a gateway to recognizing and understanding some key psychosocial aspects of disability.

Recognizing and Trying to Understand Disability

How should disabled people regard the nature of their disabilities, whether they are physical, cognitive, emotional, intellectual, psychological, or some combination thereof? In turn, how should nondisabled people construe the experience of disability, a state about which they observe and infer rather than know? One of the overarching goals underlying the creation of the foundational principles was to help disabled and nondisabled people both recognize and understand the experience of disability. To do so, both groups can become aware of the social psychological issues that influence how people perceive disability, sometimes in an open-minded manner and other times tempered by social biases (Dunn, 2018).

A SOCIAL PSYCHOLOGY OF DISABILITY: BASIC AND BRIEF

People's social lives are largely driven by construal—that is, how they currently view themselves and their environments (Wilson, 2022). We may know (or think we know) our individual social experiences accurately (e.g., having fun at a party, being sad when a holiday ends), but our knowledge of other people's experience is always indirect, uncertain, and even unknown. We can speculate about or infer what someone is thinking or feeling, but we have no way of knowing whether our assessment is correct or flat-out wrong. Of course, we can ask someone what their experience is like, but we often do not feel the need to do so because we trust our observations of their behavior and our own (presumed similar) lived experience. Alternatively, our social inferences about others may be too personal, invasive, or even awkward, or much too private, so that we choose not to share them even though they may still guide our thoughts, feelings, and actions toward the individuals in question.

As a result, we make *attributions* about why people behave the way they do. In other words, we gather information to form judgments—that is, ascribed qualities—about cause and effect in social life. The resulting judgments guide how we think, feel, and act toward others to understand them and to predict their intentions. Formally, social psychologists refer to this as attribution theory because people *attribute* cause and effect to the behavior of others as well as themselves (e.g., Jones et al., 1971; Heider, 1958; Malle, 2011; Ross, 1977). To begin, we will consider three sources of such social judgment: mere difference and social categorization, essentialism, and stigma.

MERE DIFFERENCE AND SOCIAL CATEGORIZATION

How does this attributional analysis matter where disability is concerned? One answer is straightforward: Any disability is perceived as a difference and any difference that people display is interesting; that is, it attracts the attention of others. Observers (primarily nondisabled people, but on occasion other disabled individuals) take note of the disability displayed by someone they encounter in some social situation. The person's *mere* difference—the disability—triggers a well-documented social categorization process, one that arbitrarily creates so-called ingroups and outgroups (Brewer & Brown, 1998; Fiske, 2005; Tajfel et al., 1971).

An ingroup comprises people who are perceived to be "like us" (or themselves); thus, a nondisabled person will see other nondisabled people as automatically members of their own ingroup, whereas a disabled person might regard other disabled individuals as members of their ingroup. Members of an ingroup tend to hold more favorable attitudes toward these presumed peers even when they have no real information about them or any social connection to them (Locksley, Ortiz, & Hepburn, 1980). At the same time, a nondisabled person will categorize a disabled person as distinct and different, thereby spontaneously categorizing them as a member of the outgroup (or "them" and "not like us"); of course, someone with a disability could also reach a similar conclusion about a nondisabled person.

Feelings toward outgroup members are less favorable even when the group assignment is completely arbitrary. Tajfel (2001), for example, famously demonstrated that people's purported preference for one abstract painter over another was sufficient to elicit this ingroup versus outgroup effect (i.e., "Since you like Klee and I like Kandinsky, we are clearly very different from one another"). What matters here is that ingroup members generally view outgroup members in monolithic terms—as much more like each other than they actually are (e.g., "All people with cerebral palsy are alike")—while treating fellow ingroup members as varied and even unique on any number of dimensions ("Everyone on the rugby team has a different undergrad major and belongs to different social organizations." Oakes, 2001; Linville & Jones, 1980). The former response is also known as the *outgroup homogeneity effect* (see, e.g., Boldry et al., 2007). The real problem, of course, is that this routine group categorization process built on perceived similarity or difference increases the likelihood that prejudice and discrimination—favoritism toward the ingroup and antipathy toward the outgroup—will occur. For present purposes, we are focused on perceived disability as a driver of potentially negative feelings or acts, but other recognized differences (e.g., gender, race, ethnicity, sexual orientation) can lead to a similar outcome.

Thus, without directed care and concentration, social categorization, like much of human cognition, is relatively automatic, even mindless (Langer, 2018). Most people give little thought to how they group others, but once they have done so, there are often consequences for those who are duly categorized, particularly since perceivers rarely revisit or revise their perceptions. One such consequence is essentialism.

ESSENTIALISM

One outcome tied to social categorization along group lines where disability is concerned is that it becomes an "either/or" proposition. A person either *is* disabled or *is not* disabled. Such all or nothing cataloging "essentializes" disability so that this one quality stands out among and above all the other qualities a person might have (Bloom, 2010; Dunn, Fisher, & Beard, 2013). In other words, to the average nondisabled observer, the presence of a disability—any sort of disability—can be defining, representing the "essence" of the target person. Why does this matter? Because essentializing a person's disability frames how that individual is perceived; all other aspects of the person—no matter how important (e.g., education, career, skills, sense of humor, athletic ability)—are overlooked so that the perceived disability regulates that and any subsequent social interactions. When meeting a person who is blind or has some degree of visual impairment, the observer is apt to focus on the person's vision regardless of whatever other qualities are present.

In other words, disabled persons are often thought of exclusively in terms of their disabilities, which may have little effect on their day-to-day existence. In fact, many disabled individuals only reflect on their disabilities when nondisabled others ask about them or when some environmental feature (or its absence) affects them (e.g., Dunn, 2015, 2019a). As we will learn, one of the goals of the foundational principles is to help people with disabilities navigate essentialism when they encounter it and to guide nondisabled persons away from drawing essentialist conclusions.

We now turn to a third aspect of the social psychology of disability—what happens when disability is seen as a stigma by others.

STIGMA

A stigma is a marker, or some noticeable attribute or identity quality that members of a culture or a particular context view in negative terms (Corrigan, 2014; Goffman, 1963). Casual observers routinely perceive disabilities to be a stigmatizing condition. The origins of stigma are no longer seen as being due to antisocial

TABLE 1.2

Six Dimensions of Stigma
Visible or concealable: Is the stigma apparent (e.g., a missing limb) or unseen (e.g., mood disorder)?
Origin/responsibility for condition: Is it a congenital, accidental, or self-inflicted stigma?
Aesthetic: Does the stigma distress or upset those who see it?
Perilous: Can the stigma be seen as contagious or even dangerous to others?
Disruptiveness: Can the stigma disrupt or even prevent communication or social interaction with others?
Course of the mark: As time passes, will the stigma change, dissipating or worsening?

Source: Adapted from Jones et al. (1984).

tendencies, punishment for some presumed transgression or sin, or maladaptive mental health; rather, such reactions are linked to normative psychological processes (Dovidio et al., 2011)—an outgrowth of the social categorization process discussed above (e.g., "like me" vs. "not like me," "foreign" vs. "familiar"; Macrae & Bodenhausen, 2001), thereby triggering problematic stereotypes, prejudicial attitudes, and the possibility of uncaring or even discriminatory behaviors.

Once recognized, a stigma can elicit an acute and powerful emotional response from an observer (e.g., anxiety, fear, upset, disgust; Dovidio et al., 2000; Jones et al., 1984). Jones and colleagues discussed six dimensions of stigma that can affect observers (see Table 1.2), though disabled persons are most likely to be stigmatized for visible disabilities (e.g., physical differences) or visible evidence that some disability is present (e.g., unusual gait or body motion; use of a cane, a walker, or a wheelchair). Unfortunately, there is considerable research revealing that nondisabled people frequently stigmatize the disabled (e.g., Corrigan, 2014; Fichten et al., 1988, 1991; Yuker, 1994).

Link and Phelan (2001) created a model highlighting five features of stigma discerned in interactions between nondisabled and disabled individuals. Initially, the stigma process starts when labels are applied to what are perceived as undesirable characteristics of the disability or disabled person. Following labels is stereotyping, where negative qualities are tied to disability differences that stand out; nondisabled perceivers might, for example, view a disabled person as helpless and needy. On occasion, of course, the stereotype is positive yet still problematic, as occurs when someone is deemed "heroic" or "inspirational" for managing to live with a disability. After labeling and stereotyping, social distancing takes place so that disabled targets are segregated or avoided; this can be an active process, as when a nondisabled person shuns one who is disabled, or it can be passive, which often happens in public settings when disabled people are seated separately—really sequestered—from the nondisabled.

In the fourth part of Link and Phelan's (2001) model, the social status of disabled individuals is reduced or even devalued, as when disabled children attend a public school but do not take classes, have recess, or share any activities with their nondisabled peers. Such exclusions reinforce presumptive (if often false) differences and imply that such social ostracism is acceptable.[1] In the fifth and final part of the model, the power differential between disabled and nondisabled people allows for intentional (e.g., hiring decisions) as well as unintentional (e.g., social events scheduled in inaccessible settings) discrimination to affect people with disabilities. For greater detail on this model, see Andrews (2020).

We will touch on the sources and consequences of such negativity, as well as what can be done about it, in subsequent chapters. These and other social biases (see Dunn, 2019a) can lead to and perpetuate ableism, the topic of the next section and an issue we will revisit throughout this book.

Ableism

Any time that disabled persons are subjected to implicit or explicit comparisons with able-bodied standards and related forms of social oppression, which can be subtle or rather direct, they are likely to be encountering ableism. Bogart and Dunn (2019a) defined *ableism* as the "stereotyping, prejudice, discrimination, and social oppression toward people with disabilities" (p. 651). Ableism can be intentional (e.g., asking a disabled person an inappropriate question about their condition, using a pejorative term—such as "retard"—in a joke) or unintentional (e.g., unknowingly staring at someone who has a facial disfigurement, praising a disabled person for performing a simple act of daily living, like grocery shopping). Ableist terms are often found in everyday discourse, too, as when someone argues that a policy is "myopic or shortsighted"; they can seem innocent or innocuous, but they are not (for a list of everyday ableist terms and alternatives, see Table 2.2).

1. Years ago, a disabled member of the entering class at my university was asked to move his wheelchair from the aisle where it was parked during a closing orientation gathering. He was told it was a fire hazard; he declined, as he would have had to move to the back of the auditorium rather than, as he pointed out, "sit with the members of my first-year class." Such indignities are all too common.

In general, ableism occurs when the intact, "whole" bodies of the nondisabled are touted as the ideal or a desired norm. As a result, disability is "cast as a diminished state of being human" (Campbell, 2001, p. 44). At times, ableism can seem to be innocent or even be a form of expressing concern, such as when a nondisabled person asks someone who is disabled whether their condition can be "fixed" or "surgically repaired." In other situations, ableism is more obvious, such as when a public concert venue is not accessible for wheelchair users, who are segregated a considerable distance from the stage. For more detailed reviews of ableism and its consequences, see Bogart and Dunn (2019b), Dunn (2024), Nario-Redmond (2020), and Peña-Guzmán and Reynolds (2019).

Ableism parallels the study of other "isms" in social psychology, such as racism, sexism, and ageism, among others. As we will see in the next chapter, disability is intersectional in that it necessarily co-occurs with many other qualities, like race, gender, ethnicity, sexual orientation, social class, and so on. Yet it is important to remember that as a quality, it tends to supersede the influence of other qualities where social perception and cognition are concerned (recall the earlier discussion of social categorization, essentialism, and stigma). Most research on ableism is found in the field of disability studies, an interdisciplinary arena that examines disability as a social, political, and cultural phenomenon akin to women's studies or African American studies (Bogart & Dunn, 2019a).

For our purposes, the foundational principles discussed in this book are a means for disabled persons to recognize, navigate, and counter ableism in their daily lives. A competing goal is for nondisabled people—including rehabilitation professionals—to reduce their ableist beliefs and to become allies by becoming familiar with and accepting of the foundational principles. Before we do so, we need to consider disability as a form of diversity, a topic and reality that will inform our review of the principles in subsequent chapters.

Precis and Prospects

After defining disability, the WHO ICF model, and the incidence of disability, this first chapter introduced the current foundational principles of rehabilitation psychology and their origins. The experience of disability was considered in terms of social psychological perspectives on disability, including three important sources of social judgment: mere difference and social categorization, essentialism, and stigma. The chapter closed with a discussion of ableism, a topic and challenge that will be returned to at many points in subsequent chapters. In the next chapter (Chapter 2), we will explore the ways in which disability represents a form of diversity. We will explore its intersectional nature and consider the importance of promoting inclusion and equity issues for people with disabilities.

THOUGHT QUESTIONS

1. What is disability or a disability? Is disability a quality of the person, the environment, or both?
2. Why is the term "handicap" or "handicapped" problematic? How does its technical meaning differ from its colloquial meaning?
3. Why is the WHO ICF model important for characterizing and understanding the experience of disability?
4. Disability is a ubiquitous condition, both globally and in the United States. Yet disabled people generally constitute a marginalized group. Why? What are some of the stressors or challenges they face in daily life?
5. How did the foundational principles come to be and to evolve? Why are they of benefit to both disabled and nondisabled persons? What are the current seven foundational principles?
6. The social psychology of disability is based in part on attribution theory. What are three sources of social judgment commonly used by nondisabled people to understand disabled people?
7. What is ableism, and why is it a problem for advancing the interests of people with disabilities and the foundational principles?

2 Disability as Diversity

THE IMPORTANCE OF INTERSECTIONALITY, EQUITY, AND INCLUSION

> I do not suffer from that common failing of judging another man by me: I can easily believe that others have qualities quite distinct from my own . . . I can conceive and believe that there are thousands of different ways of living.
>
> —Michel de Montaigne, *The Complete Essays* (1580)

SOME YEARS BACK, an article on the front page of the *New York Times* illustrated one of the social quandaries facing Americans today: navigating multiculturalism (Saulny, 2011). The piece explored how citizens described their racial or ethnic identification. To do so, the author profiled a then-young college student who was of "Peruvian, Chinese, Irish, Shawnee, and Cherokee descent" (p. A1). Based on procedure, one government department would categorize the student as "Hispanic," while another would select "Asian." The student's birth certificate, which was from the state of Maryland, made no mention of race. So, how did the student think about or define themselves? Sometimes the student reported checking "other" on such surveys, but when completing a census form, they checked each of the following options: Asian, Hispanic, Native American, and White. As you might imagine, representations of such multiculturalism—what is now more commonly or collectively referred to as

On the Foundational Principles of Rehabilitation Psychology. Dana S. Dunn, Oxford University Press.
 DOI: 10.1093/9780197785188.003.0002

"diversity"—have become even more complex and detailed, as have people's understandings of how they want to represent themselves and their identities and how they want others to both appraise and appreciate them. We will explore issues of diversity in this chapter, particularly those linked with or having implications for disability. Let's start by defining our terms.

Recognizing Diversity

Diversity is a term that is frequently used in higher education circles, popular culture, government, and business settings. It is revered by some and, in complicated political climates, questioned or occasionally even reviled by others. Admittedly, the term can mean different things to different people in different contexts. It is probably best to begin with a simple definition of diversity and then consider how it applies to people and, for our purposes, the field of psychology and its interest in improving the lives of people with disabilities.

At base, "diversity" refers to the existence of variety and difference. In human contexts, diversity is the practice of attracting and engaging people from dissimilar social, cultural, and ethnic backgrounds who also represent different races, genders, and sexual orientations, among other possible factors, including disability. One way to articulate a goal for diversity is to make the world a more inclusive place by promoting fairness and human rights and treating all people with dignity (see Chapter 8 for a detailed discussion of the latter). Diversity also entails equity and inclusion, two topics we will discuss later in this chapter.

Within the field of psychology and the work done by psychologists as practitioners, researchers, and educators, the American Psychological Association (APA, 2021; see also APA, 2017, 2023) outlines diversity as an essential component in any framework for examining equity, diversity, and inclusion (EDI) issues. More specifically, the APA sought to reform its own policies and procedures tied to matters of diversity, as well as those embedded in the field of psychology and in the wider society (both in the United States and globally). To achieve the latter, four domains received attention: advocacy, education, practice, and science. To advance this agenda where disability is concerned, disabled people must be viewed as representing diversity and their own culture.

DISABILITY AS DIVERSITY AND A SOURCE OF CULTURE

Disability is a form of diversity (e.g., Andrews, 2020; Dunn, 2009; Dunn, Fisher, & Beard, 2013; Dunn & Hammer, 2014; Olkin, 2002). Gill (1995), for example, argued that people with disabilities constitute a distinct culture, one that has endured prejudice and discrimination like that foisted on other groups in the United States, such as women, gays and lesbians, and people of color (e.g., Longmore & Umansky, 2001). Gill outlined four primary functions of disability culture that allow it to flourish and grow: fortification, unification, communication, and recruitment.

Fortification

Fortification entails the energy, strength, and endurance that develops due to a shared sense of purpose in the disability community. Fortification affords disabled people the opportunity to combat subtle and obvious oppression and to advocate for equal rights and economic equality. The heterogeneity of disabled groups allows different alliances to form as needed to tackle longstanding and emerging challenges.

Unification

At the same time that the heterogeneity of disability is acknowledged, it should be remembered that historically a hierarchy of stigma has existed, where some disabilities have been perceived to be less negative (e.g., a physical disability) than others (e.g., an intellectual disability). The result of such implicit stigma ranking was a splintering of relations among various disability groups due to the adoption—or worse, acceptance—of externally oppressive views (Mackelprang & Salsgiver, 2016). By organizing and seeking a common purpose, members of disability culture can unify to seek communal support and to pursue shared goals, which in turn promotes a sense of belongingness and the pursuit of mutual destiny.

Communication

One frequently overlooked aspect of life with a disability is that it is all too easy to be isolated from others who identify as disabled. Moreover, some people have congenital disabilities, while others acquire them later in life through accident or disease. And we should not ignore the fact that as people age, they may acquire health conditions that technically qualify them as disabled. As a result, fostering connection and interaction among disabled people is important so that exposure to disability culture's arts, rituals, symbols, language, social justice, and activism concerns and the like, can happen. Naturally, the evolution of technology and the internet have helped a great deal to allow for communication enabling disabled individuals to find one another, thereby signaling "to each other who we are as a distinct people" (Gill, 1995, p. 17).

Recruitment

Disability culture advances only when disabled people are enlisted to change the dominant narratives about disability, including those characterizing disability as "tragic" or linked to "suffering and pity" or, in some cases, "virtue and heroism" (as we will see in later chapters, overly positive narratives can be just as problematic). In the past, recruitment was often initiated by nondisabled people who were interested in ameliorating the medical aspects of disability, as in charities designed to advance research aimed at cures or to support families with disabled children. In contrast, contemporary disability culture is concerned with shifting the narrative toward embracing and celebrating the distinctive qualities found in the disabled community. To do so, welcoming younger and recently disabled people to join the community becomes an important goal.

The late disability lawyer, activist, and author Harriet McBryde Johnson (2003; see also 2005) countered the pervasive and familiar negative narrative that disabled people are worse off than nondisabled people. When she did so, she evoked disability as both diversity and a cultural resource:

> Are we "worse off"? I don't think so. Not in any meaningful sense. There are too many variables. For those of us with congenital conditions, disability shapes all we are. Those disabled later in life adapt. We take constraints that no one would choose and build rich and satisfying lives within them. We enjoy pleasures other people enjoy, and pleasures peculiarly our own. We have something the world needs. (p. 79)

For more detailed discussions regarding the breadth and depth of disability culture, please consult Gill (1987, 1995) and Andrews (2020). We now consider a model for understanding disability as both a form of diversity and a distinct culture.

THE DIVERSITY MODEL OF DISABILITY

A variety of models are available for describing the complexities linking people, their disabilities, and particular psychosocial outcomes at the personal and societal levels (Andrews, 2017; Wang et al., 2006). Following our review of disability as a source of diversity and culture, it makes sense to consider the diversity model of disability in this chapter. We will touch on some of the older models (e.g., moral model, medical model, social model) in subsequent chapters. The diversity model (which is occasionally referred to as the minority model) focuses on the sociopolitical aspects of disability (Altman, 2001). This model emerged from scholarship grounded in disability studies, where disability is portrayed as values-based and a core source of identity tied to diversity and culture (Andrews et al., 2013). To that end, disability represents an individual difference factor along the normal continuum of diversity—yet, as we will shortly learn, it is rarely understood to be a form of diversity. The model posits that the great obstacles that disabled individuals encounter are ableist attitudes and behaviors (recall Chapter 1). It also strongly endorses disability pride (Olkin, 2002), which is often connected to the disability in question (such as Deaf pride) as well as the use of identity-first language (e.g., disabled person) instead of person-first constructions (e.g., person with a disability; we will explore the importance and nuances of disability-related language shortly; see also Dunn & Andrews, 2015).

We now turn to whether, why, and how disabled people constitute a minority group.

DO DISABLED PEOPLE REPRESENT THE LARGEST MINORITY GROUP?

One of the unusual and generally overlooked aspects of disability is this fact: Disabled people constitute the largest minority group in the United States.[1] Yet if you asked a random citizen on the street to name the nation's largest minority group, it is highly unlikely they would do so correctly. Why? Possibly for a few reasons. First, people are used to thinking of minority groups in terms of race or ethnicity, and possibly gender. After those groupings, they may mention sexual orientation—if only because so many different and distinct labels have emerged in recent years (e.g., LGBTQ+, cisgender, pansexual). They are less likely to point to religion, social class (or socioeconomic status [SES]), or education (about 44% of US adults aged 25 and older hold some type of college degree, rendering them a minority for at least the time being; Bryant, 2023), among other factors that sociologists or demographers routinely consider.

Second—and perhaps most tellingly—most people do not consider disability to be a quality that marks or defines a minority group. Historically, disability was rarely discussed in psychology courses or curricula, a fact that has led many scholars to label people with disabilities an "invisible" minority (e.g., Asch, 1988). If people did consider disability an indicator of minority group status, they would quickly realize that the disability community is heterogenous; as noted in Chapter 1, disability comes in many forms, such as sensory, intellectual, physical, psychiatric, or linked to a chronic health condition. And, as we know, some disabilities are visible, and others not. Add to this list some newer forms of disability that qualify, such as people who identify

1. It is likely that this is true globally, as well.

as neurodiverse, including those with autism. Such individuals are not neurotypical (a synonym for being nondisabled in some contexts).

Third, as already mentioned in Chapter 1, essentialism leads observers to focus on disability as a salient quality. All other aspects that a given disabled person presents are usually ignored. And a group of people with the same type of disability are viewed as being like one another—that is, in homogeneous terms—even though such comparisons make no sense, as each person may experience the given disability somewhat differently and to a lesser or greater degree. Of course, the key factor that people miss when thinking about disability is that it is also linked with intersectionality.

Intersectionality and Disability

The term "intersectionality" seems relatively new, though it has been around since it was coined by Kimberlé Crenshaw (1989), a legal scholar who drew attention to the systemic exclusion experienced by Black women. Since then, the term "intersectionality" is understood to outline the ways that existing systems of inequality linked to race, gender, sexual orientation, ethnicity, gender identity, disability, social class, and other areas of discrimination *intersect*. The interconnectedness of these social and political categories leads to singular dynamics and effects perpetuating interdependent systems of disadvantage, as well as those allowing for opportunity and privilege—generally for majority group members (e.g., males, White people, upper- and upper-middle-class individuals, nondisabled persons).

In more practical terms, disabled people also simultaneously present other qualities tied to their identities, including race, gender expression, sexual orientation, ethnicity, and so on. Hence, collectively, disabled people represent the "largest minority" group due to the other intersectional qualities they possess. And as noted in Chapter 1, disabled persons around the world and in the United States experience considerable challenges where accessibility, income, education, jobs, and careers, among other matters, are concerned. Very often, these challenges are due to established patterns of stigmatization, prejudice, and discrimination, only some of which is recognized or addressed (more subtle or "benign bigotry" continues; see Anderson, 2010).

The practical consequences of intersectionality are important for nondisabled as well as disabled people. Unless prompted to reflect otherwise, the former are likely to ignore other factors besides a person's disability, as this quality generally overrides the importance of all the others (recall the discussion of essentialism in Chapter 1). Disabled people, on the other hand, may value their disability identity (see Chapter 5) while also thinking of themselves in terms of additional intersectional connections. As one of my colleagues, Erin Andrews, explained in the preface to her book, *Disability as Diversity*,

> The perceptions in this book are mine alone, as are any mistakes or misconstructions. I have tried to present a balanced viewpoint, but the limitations of my own experience and my biases as an upper middle-class, highly educated, White, heterosexual, physically disabled, cisgender woman should be noted. (Andrews, 2020, p. xiii)

Few disabled people are likely to "spell out" their intersectional qualities so directly in daily life, but the influence of these qualities on how they think, feel, behave, and navigate their social worlds is nonetheless present and should not be overlooked.

A related and important consideration is how these intersectional qualities impact the health and well-being of anyone who is disabled. As Bowleg (2012) wrote,

> I consider the core tenets of intersectionality most relevant to public health to be as follows: (1) social identities are not independent and unidimensional but multiple and intersecting, (2) people from multiple historically oppressed and marginalized groups are the focal or starting point, and (3) multiple social identities at the micro level (i.e., intersections of race, gender, and SES) intersect with macrolevel structural factors (i.e., poverty, racism, and sexism) to illustrate or produce disparate health outcomes. (p. 1268)

We will discuss quite a few of these intersectional health qualities in later chapters in this book. We now consider equity and inclusion issues related to disability.

Equity, Inclusion, and Disability

In current discussions of diversity, the concepts of equity and inclusion are usually considered in tandem—hence the popular acronyms DEI and EDI. Equity occurs when diverse individuals receive resources that they need to navigate their particular circumstances in ways leading to desired outcomes (e.g., health, employment, education) (APA, 2024b). Though related to one another, please note that equity is not the same thing as "equality," a term that refers to situations where people receive the same rights and opportunities. When equality is present, everyone receives the same outcome, whereas equity provides each person with the level of outcome that will be most beneficial for them individually. Consider providing accommodations for learning disabled students in classroom settings: Giving everyone the same accommodation (e.g., the same amount of additional time to complete an exam, allowing a writing assignment to be submitted late with no penalty) may not be helpful to all students. Providing equitable accommodations would mean that some disabled students would receive more additional time to complete an exam or paper than others due to their respective disabilities. When equity is in play, everyone in each situation receives the amount or level they individually need to succeed.

Where disability is concerned, equity often entails issues of social justice, which entails offering a fair balance when the sharing of opportunities, wealth, and privileges in a society affords recognition and protection of all individuals' rights. Although legislation, such as the Americans with Disabilities Act (1990), has promoted the importance of attending to the civil rights and needs of disabled persons, acute challenges remain that can threaten the welfare of the disability community. During the start of the COVID-19 pandemic in the winter and spring of 2020, for example, health care providers around the world were overwhelmed by people who were infected with the virus. Deaths skyrocketed, particularly among older people and those with various comorbidities. Effective vaccines to combat the virus did not appear until the spring of 2021. Some, but by no means all, disabilities put people at higher risk for infection and medical complications. Disabled people living in institutional settings, such as group or nursing homes, as well as assisted living facilities, were at high risk due to the confining nature of the settings, which allowed the virus to spread quickly. It has also become clear that disabled individuals experienced mental health needs during the COVID-19 pandemic, but frequently they encountered barriers to obtaining the necessary services due to disability bias and lack of disability competence training among professional medical staff (Manning et al., 2023). In Chapter 9, we will review how the demand for relevant medical equipment (e.g., ventilators) outstripped available supplies and the shortages led to triage guidelines, so that some patients were prioritized over others, who received no aid (Andrews et al., 2021). Disabled people were understandably alarmed that they might be seen as a lower priority than nondisabled people, which would constitute an example of medical ableism (recall Chapter 1).

What about issues of inclusion? The term "inclusion" is used to create an environment (e.g., social, workplace, recreational) that provides "affirmation, celebration, and appreciation of different approaches, styles, perspectives, and experiences" (APA, 2024b). Inclusive environments are welcoming to diverse individuals because people are accepting of and interested in learning about their worldviews. Thus, regarding disability, an inclusive community would be one that promoted awareness and acceptance of the perspectives of its disabled members.

Inclusion can mean many things, but one key arena that promotes it is the way in which people understand and use language to navigate diversity.

Inclusiveness and Language

Language is powerful: Some words can be used to praise or honor individuals or groups, and others can marginalize or even harm them. How can language be more inclusive? Generally, one way to make communications with others more inclusive is by choosing appropriately respectful terms and calling people (or referring to them) by what they call themselves or prefer to be called (APA, 2023). An important caveat is that language evolves, sometimes rapidly, which means that terms that were once acceptable may no longer be deemed appropriate or sensitive. And words that work well in one context can be unacceptable or even offensive in another setting; care, sensitivity, and attention to context and culture can matter a great deal. As we have already learned, due to intersectionality, people possess (potentially) multiple identities that are influenced by a variety of social forces, including oppressive ones and those that provide certain privileges. It is in the interests of practitioners, researchers, educators, and students of psychology to try to remain aware of changes and additions to inclusive language.

Besides choosing spoken words carefully, writers will want to rely on inclusive language, as well. In addition to the *Inclusive Language Guide* (APA, 2023), you may want to refer to the *Publication Manual of the American Psychological Association* (APA, 2020), which contains guidance on how to write about people and to represent their diverse qualities appropriately (additionally, the APA website often includes updates concerning the use of inclusive language in written and spoken communication; www.apa.org). In the sections that follow, we review some of the guidelines that are most appropriate for writing using EDI language tied to disability. For specific recommendations regarding writing (or speaking, for that matter) about age, body size and weight, neurodiversity, race, ethnicity, culture, sexual orientation, gender diversity, socioeconomic status, and culturally appropriative and pejorative language, please consult APA (2020, 2023).

PERSON-FIRST AND IDENTITY-FIRST LANGUAGE

For decades, Division 22 (Rehabilitation Psychology) of the APA advocated for acceptance and use of what is known as *person-first language* to refer to disability, as did the APA itself, particularly in its policies and publications, including books and scholarly journals. The goal of person-first constructions was to "put the person first, before the disability" to emphasize the former rather than the latter. Hence, psychologists were trained to say or write about a "person with an amputation" rather than an "amputee," the assumption being that the latter label was monolithic and objectifying

(Dunn, 2015; Dunn & Andrews, 2015; see also Andrews et al., 2022). Using terms like "amputee," "diabetic," or even "disabled" was seen as being no different than depending on labels that segregated people into racial, ethnic, and other groupings, where doing so reduced or even overlooked individual differences among the group members (e.g., Allport, 1954; Wiley et al., 2012). Indeed, such homogenization can promote stereotypes, loss of individuality, and potential victimization (e.g., Dunn & Elliott, 2005, 2008; Wright, 1991); recall the discussion of social categorization ("us vs.us them") in Chapter 1.

As time passed, however, both disability culture advocates and scholars in disabilities studies began to question the logic, legitimacy, and social impact of person-first language: To wit, they claimed that it was hiding disability and implying such conditions were pejorative in nature (e.g., Brueggemann, 2013; Davis, 2013; Goodley, 2011; Longmore, 2003; Shapiro, 1994). They advocated for researchers, educators, practitioners, students, and the lay public to both promote and accept the use of *identity-first language* (e.g., disabled people). Disabled people themselves argued that their disability was an important part of their identities and should therefore become the focus. As Brueggmann (2013) argued,

> Disability is not a state of bodily impairment, inadequacy, failing misfortune, or excess—that it is not about marking the things gone "wrong" with the body. Rather, disability, as it is conceived in disability studies is a culturally composed (and shared) narrative of the body . . . a study of the unequal distribution of power, material and economic resources, and status (class, etc.) within both social and architectural environments. (p. 283)

This social and psychological sea change allowed disabled individuals and groups to "claim" disability as a reality and to present it as a source of pride. Such claiming is a way to value disability so that others—including family members, peers, employers, educators, and medical professionals—recognize that the disabled person is choosing their identity instead of allowing others to do so for them (Brueggemann, 2013). Identity-first constructions suggest agency, autonomy, and choice. As one psychologist colleague was quoted in Dunn and Andrews (2015, p. 257), "I am absolutely not a 'person with autism.' It's [the autism] not detachable." This repatriation of once avoided or even forbidden terms is like the way LGBTQ+ activists claimed the word "queer" in their fight for civil rights, including same-sex marriage.[2]

2. Within the disability community, some activists have claimed once-insulting slang and epithets (e.g., crip, gimp, para) and used it in written and spoken discourse for protest and rallying purposes. This is an example of an ingroup phenomenon advancing social causes; however, under no circumstances should nondisabled people use such terms in any medium or for any purpose (see also Table 2.1).

Does this mean that person-first language should be discarded? No, not at all. The disability community meets under a "big tent," and there are members within it who prefer person-first language over identity-first constructions. The best approach—again—is to discern what a person or people in question prefer. If you are unsure, ask, and if you cannot do so, using person-first language may be the best route. In terms of written works, using a mixture of person-first and identify-first is an acceptable way to proceed unless the individuals being discussed prefer one over the other. For more detail on these issues, see Dunn and Andrews (2015), Andrews et al. (2022), the *APA Publication Manual* (APA, 2020), and the *APA Inclusive Language Guide* (2023).

LANGUAGE CHOICES FOR DISABILITY

What are some examples of appropriate language for discussing disability and people with disabilities? Table 2.1 shows some examples of terms that are designed to reflect disability culture and its diversity. Both person-first and identity-first constructions are presented. Note that the left column in the table lists terms that should be avoided, while the right column lists recommended alternatives that can be used. These entries are not exhaustive, but the examples can suggest ways to craft novel constructions as needed. As always, context matters, and language does evolve; it's quite possible that some of the terms in Table 2.1 that are currently apropos may not be so in the future. Rehabilitation practitioners, researchers, and educators should try to remain abreast of relevant language trends to best serve their clients and their families.

Table 2.2 lists examples of problematic ableist terms and phrases that appear in everyday language. Some entries are so commonplace in our culture's discourse that readers may be surprised to learn that they are prejudicial and can cause offense—but they are and they can. It can be a challenge to stop using familiar idioms, and it is probably easier to do so when writing than when speaking. Still, to advance the rights of disabled people and to promote diversity, equity, and inclusion, the effort is warranted, especially by professionals who work with disabled individuals and their families.

In addition, deciding to stop using words and phrases like those shown in Table 2.2 is a first step toward avoiding committing *microaggressions* when speaking or writing about disability. Microaggressions are short, often subtle verbal or nonverbal, behavior-based, and situational humiliations that convey negative attitudes or feelings toward someone who is "different" (Sue et al., 2007). Some microaggressions are intentional others are unintentional (APA, 2017). The chief problem is that their negative effects can accumulate across time, thereby leading to psychosocial

TABLE 2.1

Some Disability Terms to Avoid with Recommended Options

Terms to be avoided	Recommended options
Person with deafness	Deaf person*
Hearing-impaired person	Hard-of-hearing person, person who is hard-of-hearing
Person who is hearing impaired	Person with hearing loss
Person with blindness	Blind person, person who is blind
Person with deafness and blindness	Deaf-Blind person, Deaf person with low vision
	Person who is deaf with low vision
Special needs	Disabled person
Differently abled	Person with a disability
Multiabled	Person who has a disability
Physically challenged	
Mentally challenged	Person with an intellectual disability
Mentally retarded	Child with a congenital disability
Handi-capable	Child with a birth impairment
Handicapped	Physically disabled person
Suffering with . . . (condition or disability)	Person with a physical disability
Mentally ill	Person with a mental disorder
	Person with a mental illness
	Person living with a mental health condition
Wheelchair bound person	Wheelchair user
Confined to a wheelchair	Person who uses a wheelchair
Cripple	
Invalid	
Gimp	
AIDS victim	Person with AIDS
HIV patient	Person with HIV
	HIV-positive person
Brain-damaged	Person with a traumatic brain injury (TBI)
Defective	Person with a mental disorder
Nuts	Person with a mental illness

TABLE 2.1 *Continued*

Terms to be avoided	Recommended options
Crazy	Person living with a mental illness
Alcoholic	Person with alcohol use disorder
Addict	Person with substance use disorder

*The Deaf community specifically advocates using the capital D in the word "Deaf."
Source: Adapted from APA (2023)

harm. Use of the term "micro" does not mean the transgression is tiny or barely noticeable; instead, it means that the aggressive act occurs on a person-to-person, or micro, level, as when a nondisabled person sighs audibly because a disabled individual seems to be taking too long to get into an elevator. Coined by Pierce and colleagues (1977), microaggressions come in various forms, including microinsults, microassaults, and microinvalidations (Sue et al., 2007; Sue & Spanierman, 2020). Vigilance and self-reflection, of course, can help combat microaggressions, but concrete guidance for steps and dialogues that targets of microaggressions, their allies, and bystanders can use—so-called microinterventions—are available (see Sue et al., 2019, 2021). Rehabilitation practitioners and educators may be especially interested in these antiaggression approaches for their work with and for disabled clients.

To close this section of the chapter, I consider it important to reveal some sociocultural considerations surrounding the use of the term "disability." We know that despite the importance of language's effects on attitudes and beliefs toward disabled people, there have been some attempts to avoid using the term "disability." Reasons vary, but one illustrative case should be sufficient to clarify concerns, including those potentially leading to unintended consequences.

An article by Andrews et al. (2019) drew attention to a committee's decision involving disability that went awry. At the 2018 APA Annual Convention, a resource room providing accommodations and other disability-related needs for attendees was intentionally renamed the Multi-Abled Resource Room to remove the word "disability." The Committee on Disability Issues in Psychology (CDIP) decided on the name change to encourage greater utilization of the resource room.[3] The committee's reasoning was that the resource room would be seen as more inclusive toward APA attendees who could benefit from it but who also did not identify themselves as being disabled. Further, by eliminating "disability" from the name, any "users" would not be "outed," and therefore they would be protected from any potential

3. I was a member of the CDIP from 2013 thru 2015.

TABLE 2.2

Some Ableist Terms to Avoid in Everyday Discourse and Recommended Options

Terms to be avoided	Recommended options
Stand up for	Support
	Champion
Turn a blind eye to	Ignore
	Refuse to notice
Be myopic or shortsighted	Ignore
	Miss
Have a blind spot for	Show unconscious bias
Blind review	Anonymous review
Blind coding	Masked review
	Masked coding
Color blind	Deuteranomaly, achromatopsia (or other type of color-vision deficiency)
	Color-vision deficiency
Fall on deaf ears	Be willfully ignorant
	Be deliberately ignorant
Tone deaf	Insensitive
	Out of context
Midget	Little person
	Person of small stature
	Dwarf
	Having dwarfism (Little People of America, 2021)
Lame	Boring
	Mundane
	Uncool
Lend your voice	Support
Everyone should have a voice (in)	Everyone should have input in this matter
Make your voice heard	Express your perspective/opinion
Able-bodied	Nondisabled

Source: Adapted from APA (2023)

discrimination. There have been many attempts to employ euphemisms in place of the word "disability," such as "differently abled," "special needs," "handicapable," and "physically challenged" (Hojati, 2012; Marks, 1999). These and other euphemisms are meant to downplay the negative associations tied to disability and to focus on the assets of disabled individuals, yet they create problems of their own (see Table 2.2).

The name change triggered much debate among disabled psychologists regarding language use and language choices, so much so that the discussion was broadened to include Division 22 (Rehabilitation Psychology). Conversations with the APA leadership ensued after the 2018 convention, and a decision was made to return the word "disability" to the name of the resource room at subsequent national conventions.

As Andrews and colleagues (2019) explained, while they were relieved and gratified by the eventual outcome, they took to social media and created the #SaytheWord movement. Their goal was a straightforward one: to embrace disability identity and to encourage others, including nondisabled allies, to do the same. At the same time, the #SaytheWord movement hoped to get nondisabled people to stop trying to avoid and replace disability as a source of identity. Disability identity, which will be discussed in more detail in Chapter 5, refers to having positive or beneficial self-beliefs about one's own disability and having favorable ties to other members of the disability community (Dunn & Burcaw, 2013; Forber-Pratt et al., in press; Gill, 1997; Olkin & Pledger, 2003). Any attempt to erase use of the word "disability" is an affront to those promoting positive disability identities, as diminished awareness of or even loss of the word could lead to adverse sociopolitical outcomes, including the reduction or elimination of public services and supports for people with disabilities. Quite simply, the #SaytheWord movement wanted to make nondisabled people become more culturally competent about disability.

Acquiring Cultural Competence

One of the goals of this chapter is to provide readers with a sufficient understanding of cultural competence tied to disability matters so that they can better appreciate and use the foundational principles presented in the remainder of this book in their own work. Authentic cultural competence is the deliberate development of an evolving set of attitudes, behaviors, and skills to appreciate, understand, and effectively interact with others who have diverse cultural and linguistic experiences, identities, and beliefs. For present purposes, we are interested in the acquisition of cultural competence appropriate to understanding disability, people with disabilities, various subcultures within the disability community, and disability culture more generally (e.g., Andrews, 2020; Andrews et al., 2013; Dunn, 2015; Dunn & Andrews, 2015; Gill, 1995). By developing cultural competence, professionals in rehabilitation psychology and related fields—practitioners, researchers, educators, students, and interns, among others—will be more reflective in their private, professional, and public lives. Cultural competence—and cultural humility—can help them navigate the diverse social communities of disability and improve their relationships and outcomes in educational, professional, work, and community settings.

Precis and Prospects

We explored why disability is an often overlooked or even ignored form of diversity. Disabled people are often called the forgotten "minority group"—when collectively they represent arguably the largest minority group due to the intersectional nature of disability. That is, disabled people present numerous other factors that tie them to various social, demographic, and identity groupings; one's disabled status is also connected to and consequential for issues of race, ethnicity, gender identity, gender expression, sexual identity, sexual expression, religious beliefs, and social class, among other factors. Attention to intersectionality and disability is important for understanding inclusion and equity issues, as well as using appropriate language (i.e., person-first or identity-first constructions) for speaking or writing about disability. Learning these nuances can promote effective cultural competence for working with and advocating for disabled people and their communities. In the next chapter (Chapter 3), we review the social psychological importance of the first foundational principle, the so-called person-environment relation. As we will see, environmental constraints usually matter more than personality factors where living with a disability is concerned.

THOUGHT QUESTIONS

1. How should diversity be defined? Why is advocating for diversity an important goal for psychology?
2. Why and how is disability a form of diversity? How do disabled persons represent a distinct culture? What four factors did Gill (1995) advance as important for disability culture?
3. Describe the diversity model of disability and its components.
4. Why and how can disabled people represent the largest minority group in the United States? What is intersectionality, and what role does it play in supporting this claim?
5. How do issues of equity and inclusion affect disability and disabled people?
6. Why is learning inclusive language for disability so important? Why are some disabled professionals and activists concerned about the erasure of the word "disability"?
7. Why is acquiring cultural competence important for interacting with and advocating for people with disabilities?

3 Principle 1

THE PERSON AND THE ENVIRONMENT RELATION

Foundational Principle 1: The Person-Environment Relation

Attributions about people with disabilities tend to focus on presumed dispositional rather than available situational characteristics. Environmental constraints usually matter more than personality factors to living with a disability.

> Our behavior is purposeful; we live in a psychological reality or living space that includes not only those parts of our physical and social environment that are important to us but also imagined states that do not currently exist.
>
> —Kurt Lewin, *Resolving Social Conflicts* (1997)

> Human beings, viewed as behaving systems, are quite simple. The apparent complexity of our behavior over time is largely a reflection of the complexity of the environment in which we find ourselves.
>
> —Herbert A. Simon, *The Sciences of the Artificial* (1969, p. 53)

This chapter examines the first foundational principle, which is known as the *person-environment relation.* Among other issues, we will be interested in exploring why attributions about disability—judgments, perceptions, expectations, suspicions, any conclusion, really—generally involve dispositional (i.e., personality-related) qualities instead of available situational influences (i.e., environmental factors or

On the Foundational Principles of Rehabilitation Psychology. Dana S. Dunn, Oxford University Press.
 DOI: 10.1093/9780197785188.003.0003

constraints). As we will learn, in practice, the latter usually matter more than do personality factors to living life with a disability. We will attempt to answer an important question: Why do nondisabled people miss or overlook environmental constraints that affect disabled people?

Let's begin with an all-too-common event: Promising but not delivering physically accessible spaces for disabled individuals. As already acknowledged, the built world we inhabit was not designed with disability in mind. As civil rights for persons with disabilities have advanced, so has the realization that matters of accessibility and egress are important when designing structures that anyone should be able to use with relative ease. Yet it still comes as a surprise—or perhaps a shock—when a public venue is not necessarily navigable for people with disabilities. Unfortunately, we do not lack examples to illustrate relevant problems.

In 2021, the Emmy Awards announced that the presentation stage would be more accessible so that any disabled actors, writers, or directors would be able to mount it with no difficulty. One wheelchair user, the codirector of the acclaimed film *Crip Camp* (Newman & LaBrecht, 2020), James LaBrecht, planned to use it during the ceremony (Lopez, 2021). Yet during the awards program, no ramp or other structural aid to access the stage was present, and LaBrecht called out the problem on Twitter (now rebranded as X), complaining that the CBS Network and the Television Academy lied to him and to others about the stage's accessibility. By now, you should not be surprised by such incidents of everyday ableism, and yet there is something odd about promising and promoting disability accessibility but then failing to deliver it (especially when the director of a film about disability was involved in the proceedings). Ableism was clearly present here, but there are other layers of meaning to explore. We need to examine the person-environment relation and its implications in greater detail.

Kurt Lewin and the Person-Environment Relation

Like many German intellectuals, the social psychologist, Kurt Lewin (1890–1947) arrived in the United States in the 1930s as Germany was falling under the sway of the Nazi party (Marrow, 1977). The Gestalt psychology movement then popular in his native country's intellectual life shaped his psychological perspective, including his well-known field theory (Lewin, 1935). This theory posited that human behavior results from individuals' current perceptions of themselves and their environment, which was articulated in his well-known formula, behavior $(B) = f($person $[P]$, environment $[E])$, or "behavior is a function of the person and the environment."

Lewin emphasized that this did not necessarily entail the *objective* characteristics of the person and situation, such as the individual's personality traits (e.g., extraversion, optimism) or any environment enticements (e.g., available rewards—money, food—for performing certain actions). Rather, Lewin was interested primarily in the person's *perceptions* of themselves and their current environment, defining the "life space" as "the person and the psychological environment as it exists [for the person]" (Lewin, 1951/1997, p. 210).

Practically speaking, this formulation means that how people perceive their environments (i.e., their "situations" in everyday parlance) influences their subjective experience and how they subsequently behave (Ross & Nisbett, 1991). Thus, for example, a highly extroverted lawyer is likely to control their expressiveness in public settings by waiting to be called upon before addressing the courtroom and to take turns asking questions. In other public settings—say, at a raucous university basketball game—the same lawyer can shout and cheer along with the crowd without worrying about the implications of their public demeanor. So, how individuals react to social stimuli is predicated on the idea that psychological characteristics attributed to nature (e.g., personality factors) or those linked to nurture (e.g., roles we inhabit, expectations we learn, existing norms) cannot provide complete answers to questions about the origins of behavior. Sometimes the influence of the situation is sufficient to explain what behavior occurs or does not occur (courtroom decorum or the zeal of a sports fan). To truly explain witnessed behavior, we need to look at the *interaction* between the person and their perceived environment (i.e., $P \times E$); sometimes the situation overrides the influence of personal factors, and other times not.

Lewin's person-environment relation and field theory (Lewin, 1935) helped to shape subsequent models of disability, notably the conceptual pathways of the WHO (2001) International Classification of Functioning, Disability, and Heath (ICF) model that was discussed in Chapter 1 (see also Bentley et al., 2019; Dunn, 2016; Dunn et al., 2013). Wright (1960, 1983) championed the roles of environmental (E) characteristics, personal (P) factors, and the importance of $P \times E$ interactions. Trieschmann (1987) later broadened the Wrightian view of the $P \times E$ interaction to also include a role for biological-organic factors (O), which can affect functioning and health, recasting the Lewinian equation as $B = f\ (P, O, E)$ (see, for example, Chan et al., 2009).

Table 3.1 lists examples of personal and environmental factors. To be sure, the importance of particular personal factors will vary culturally and geographically so that they may interact clearly and consistently with some environments but then not with others (and vice versa; see Chan et al., 2009). Environmental factors (see the bottom of Table 3.1) constitute external factors that populate the physical, social, and

TABLE 3.1

Examples of Personal and Environmental Factors Affecting Behavior

Personal Factors
Gender identity
Age
Existing health conditions
Coping style with stress
Social/socioeconomic class (SES)
Educational attainment
Profession
Past experiences
Character style (e.g., resilience)
Personality
Meaning in life
Environmental Factors
Technological products and equipment
Natural environment and human-initiated interventions to change the environment
Support and relationships (e.g., animals, attendants, aids)
Attitudes harbored by those external to the person in the situation that originate from customs, practices, ideologies, values, norms, factual beliefs, religious convictions
Services, systems, policies, rules

Note: Adapted from Chan et al. (2009) and Wehmeyer and Dunn (2022).

attitudinal aspects of the community where people live and conduct their private and public lives. Not surprisingly, the perceived environment can promote or inhibit the inclusion of disabled persons or those with chronic health conditions. As already acknowledged, some environments inhibit access for people with mobility issues, while others are designed explicitly to allow freedom of movement, with or without some assistance (e.g., cane, walker, wheelchair or powerchair, service animal, attendant). Positive attitudes from others can create welcoming settings, allowing disabled individuals to flourish within them, just as negative attitudes can rebuff or preclude their full participation.

Rehabilitation practitioners will want to reflect on how some of the personal factors listed in Table 3.1 could play a role in a therapeutic intervention. Further, they may wish to consider how one or more of these personal factors might interact with a client's perceived environment (see the factors listed in the bottom of Table 3.1). In other words, could the presence of a person-environment interaction be helpful in developing a treatment plan for a particular client? Alternatively, could the interaction between some personal and environmental factors inhibit such treatment?

We now consider how a disabled person's behavior can lead observers to render detailed personality judgments.

Behavior as Presumptively Revealing of Personality

Although the person-environment relation highlighted both factors, Lewin noted that observers tend to ignore the impact of situations or environmental factors on behavior. Instead, they are more likely to pay attention to qualities that are attributable to the person, like presumed dispositional (i.e., personality) characteristics (Nisbett, 1980). Why does this matter in general, or with particular regard to observers' judgments about disability? As Nisbett (1980, p. 111) noted, citing Heider (1958), "The layperson errs in presuming more individual consistency in behavior from one situation to another than is warranted." This outcome means that a person of interest's behavior is so salient—that is, prominent or attention-getting—that it is mostly attributed to the person and not the situational factors simultaneously being encountered.

Imagine a scenario like this one: A casual observer sees that a wheelchair user has difficulty getting seated in a car; perhaps the vehicle is too small or the moveable seats do not provide sufficient room for sitting. The observer is likely to perceive the problem as tied to the person rather than the constraints found in the environment (the design of the small car, the space available for the immoveable seats). Social perceivers routinely overlook or even discount the influences tied to the situation in favor of the person and, here, the person's disability. In other words, the disabled person and the person's behavior (here, a struggle to get into the car) become the primary focus of the observer—the context or situational effects fade into the background.

Witnesses to and participants who take part in situations like this one can reach very different conclusions concerning what happened and why. A compelling explanation for the present example is known in social psychology as the *actor/observer bias* (Jones & Nisbett, 1971). Here, the wheelchair user has the role of the *actor*, one who looks to the situation and its external qualities (e.g., psychological or physical demands of the setting, the components of the task being done, other people, or even chance elements) to explain their behavior ("This car is too small for me and I cannot move the seats in a way that will allow me to sit comfortably."). At the same time, an *observer* watching the actor's behavior is likely to explain it by appealing to some internal presumed quality linked to the actor ("His clunky wheelchair makes it difficult to get into any car.") or a dispositional characteristic ("He must be frustrated anytime he needs to go anywhere—he must be unhappy all the time."). The psychological consequence here is that actors look to their situation to explain their behavior or why it is constrained, while observers look to the actor and their perceived—and presumed—intentions or internal states to explain the latter's actions (Heider, 1958).

Based on the results of a meta-analysis, Malle (2006) argued that the actor-observer bias is a bit less robust than the evidence warrants, except perhaps on those occasions when an actor is viewed as behaving in an idiosyncratic manner. Since disability is a salient quality, one that draws observers' attention, it may often serve as being contextually distinctive—at least compared to the behavior of nondisabled individuals. Thus, observers could be likely to explain the behavior of a disabled actor as being dispositionally based. In the absence of a curb cut, for example, a wheelchair user may not be able to cross a street at a desired point. To compensate, the actor may think to themselves, "Since I cannot cross here, I'll move further down the block in search of a curb cut." A nondisabled observer, in turn, who did not know the actor, might misinterpret the actor's behavior, thinking, "Well, imagine being that helpless and not able to cross a street—why doesn't he have a companion to push his chair and lower it down into the street for him?"

When observers do focus on an actor's presumed dispositions (that is, personality traits) as more important than any situational influences, their often-erroneous inferences represent what social psychologists refer to as the *fundamental attribution error* (Ross, 1977), which is also known as *correspondence bias* (Gilbert & Malone, 1995; see also Gilbert, 1998). Thus, the aforementioned wheelchair user or any physically disabled person could have their actions explained away as representing dependence, helplessness, haplessness, awkwardness, or other possible traits tied to what they did or did not do behaviorally. Because these social judgments are made effortlessly, automatically, and more or less unconsciously, observers rarely learn if they are correct or, as we assume in many cases, biased (see, for example, Nisbett & Ross, 1980). Still, these sorts of attributions do provide observers with feelings of perceived control and a sense of predictability where understanding social encounters is concerned (for a review of other biases tied to social and rehabilitation psychology, see Dunn, 2019c).

Naive Realism: A Greater Attribution Error?

> In all matters of opinion our adversaries are insane.
>
> —Mark Twain (1899)

Mark Twain's observation may seem a bit extreme, yet most of us can identify moments when we have considered someone who disagrees with us regarding some apparent truth to be ridiculously wrong: How can they see the situation in any way but the way we ourselves do? In some of his later research, Lee Ross and his colleagues explored this phenomenon, which they referred to as "naive realism" (e.g., Pronin et al., 2002, 2004; Ross & Ward, 1996; see also Ross, 2018). *Naive realism* entails believing in an illusion of personal objectivity; that is, there is clearly only one objective reality, and we feel we recognize it and know it well because we ourselves are not biased. Indeed, naive realism encourages the perceiver to assume that reasonable people can only agree with our own judgments rather than finding fault with them. Yet experience tells us that such strong convictions can nonetheless trigger misunderstanding, mistrust, and even conflict if we cannot persuade others to accept our conclusions. If they refuse to accept our insights, then they are being obstinate, unreasonable, and possibly even irrational, just as Twain observed over 100 years ago.

In an article on the development of his research interests across his career, Ross (2018) suggested that naive realism represents the *truly* fundamental attribution error in that the illusion of personal objectivity has decided consequences for interpersonal and intergroup relations and interactions. To wit, if an observer assumes that a disabled person cannot be happy due to the presence of a disability, then that observer cannot entertain accounts to the contrary; any reports of supposed happiness or well-being must be false or a form of wishful thinking or even malingering. In general, many people see disability as a negative state, so *it must be so*, regardless of what the disabled person in question or their family and friends otherwise report (we review this possibility in detail in Chapter 4).

Certainly, naive realism can also incorporate the attribution errors tied to the presumed presence of personality traits as explanations for behavior. But the personal objectivity illusion goes beyond that, manifesting itself as the *false consensus effect* (we assume other people feel the same as we do; Ross et al., 1977) and *overconfidence in accurately predicting future actions and outcomes about self and others* (we *just know* what we and others will do in the fullness of time; Dunning et al., 1990; Vallone et al., 1990), among other psychosocial phenomena (see Ross, 2018 and Gilovitch & Ross, 2015 for more detailed discussions). In short, we have a *bias blind spot* whereby we see cognitive and motivational biases as much more at work in the judgments made by others than those conclusions we reach ourselves (Pronin et al., 2002). Authentic objectivity, then, at least in the eyes of human beholders, is illusory.

Clearly, the fundamental attribution error and naive realism have decided consequences where disability and disabled persons are concerned. We now turn to two biases that were discerned by rehabilitation psychologists. These biases are important for rehabilitation professionals to recognize in clinical settings, as they can influence relations with disabled clients and their families.

Fundamental Negative Bias and Labeling

The environment and factors within it are not the only influences that can be overlooked in the process of social perception. We know that negative qualities often attract more attention than positive ones, leading some social psychologists to claim that "bad is stronger than good" (Baumeister et al., 2001). For example, cataloged negative emotions outnumber positive ones by about three to one, and they tend to have a more pronounced impact on people than do positive ones. Similarly, negative impressions and stereotypes emerge faster and are more difficult to change than upbeat ones. When this happens, social observers are apt to overlook or ignore any available positive information and instead focus on and overemphasize any present negative qualities. And without sustained and conscious effort, these initially negative evaluations will remain readily available in one's cognitive arsenal for quick, uncontrolled application to our social lives (e.g., Bargh et al., 1996). And where decisions are concerned, particularly when risk is involved, losses loom larger in the minds of perceivers than do gains (a variant of the "bad is stronger than good" claim; Kahneman & Tversky, 1979).

Imagine an attractive young woman who happens to use a cane crossing a hotel lobby. She is stopped by a stranger, who blithely exclaims, "My, you are much too young and too pretty to have to use a cane!" Wright (1988) referred to reactions like these as evidence for what she called *fundamental negative bias*, which occurs when some characteristic of an object or a person attracts attention (i.e., saliency), is processed for whatever reason as being negative (i.e., value), and the context where it is operating is vague, poorly defined, or sparse (i.e., context).[1] In this instance, the negatively valanced cane is salient, just as the stranger implies that youthful and attractive individuals should not have to use such aids—but what is likely intended as a compliment is also experienced as a mild insult or a put-down (i.e., attractive individuals don't use mobility supports; recall the discussion of microaggressions in Chapter 2).

The context can influence meaning or, as Wright (1991) claimed, "The context can refer to conditions external to the perceiver or to intrapsychic predispositions of various sorts" (p. 471). Wright suggested that when these three criteria are met, then the

1. Of course, it is also possible for people to express a fundamental positive bias in their interactions with others. Such an occurrence happens when something perceived as very noticeable, favorable, and found in an ambiguous context represents a primary influence in leading an individual's future perception, cognition, and affect in positive directions (see Wright, 1988).

negative value tied to the object or person will bias subsequent perceptions, thoughts, and feelings to match its negative quality. Practically speaking, the fundamental negative bias increases the magnitude of any undesirable features people recognize as they navigate their social worlds.

When a nondisabled person encounters a disabled person, the disability automatically becomes a salient concern—whether it is physical, mental, intellectual, or some other category—so that the perceiver focuses on it, ignoring any positive information in the situation. A recent *New York Times* advice column illustrates the fundamental negative bias in action (Galanes, 2024). A parent wrote about her son, who was paralyzed years ago in a sporting accident, as someone who leads a life full of friends, a career, sporting activities, and a great deal of fun. Yet, even now, a woman friend in the parent's social circle continues to focus on the son's mobility issues with a tinge of sadness, all the while applauding the parent's "bravery" and claiming the son is "an inspiration" to others (we will discuss the problems posed by characterizing disabled individuals as "brave" or "inspiring" or the similar in Chapter 4).

As the parent put it to the advice columnist, the son is more than just his legs, so why doesn't the friend accept this reality? The columnist concurred, noting that the friend's compassion seems to have morphed into pity with a whiff of superiority, though the friend may be endlessly focused on the paralysis because she does not know how she herself would cope with this situation if a similar accident happened to her or one of her children. The columnist suggests that the parent respond directly but gently, reminding the friend that the accident happened years ago and her son—and they—have moved beyond the event to embrace the fulfilling life he leads. Pointedly, the parent was encouraged to ask the friend why the son's disability continues to resonate so much in her thoughts.

Although it was conducted for another empirical purpose, an older study by Whiteman and Lukoff (1965) illustrates the fundamental negative bias in action. Research participants were asked to read and to rate labels such as "blindness" versus "blind people" and "physical handicap" versus "physically handicapped people." (Please note that this research was conducted before person-first language [recall the discussion in Chapter 2] became widely adopted in the field of psychology—but see Dunn & Andrews, 2015.) When evaluating pairs of labels, respondents tended to rate the disabled states (e.g., blindness) much more negatively than people described as experiencing the state (e.g., blind people). Thus, blindness, physical disability, and other similar labels that singled out a condition were treated as salient, negative qualities. When labels lack a supporting context to guide judgment—say, the identification or a person or a group sharing some quality—the rating is more negative. Attaching a word like "people" or "person" provides the needed context, thereby moderating the fundamental negative bias and leading to more favorable ratings (hence the advent of person-first language).

Like the fundamental attribution error and naive realism, the fundamental negative bias is a challenge to recognize in daily life. Negatively valanced objects and people typically guide our interest, so that unless we are consciously and carefully reviewing the available factors connected to a target, we, like the overly solicitous friend described above, can ignore useful, even diagnostic, positive information that is present. We will return to examples like these in Chapter 4 when we explore the second foundational principle, the insider-outsider distinction.

We now consider a related consequence of this phenomenon, how labeling people's conditions—whether tied to disability or a chronic health condition—can lead observers to miss characteristics that distinguish people from one another.

(DE)INDIVIDUATION AND LABELING

Rehabilitation psychologists have long been concerned that one of the negative consequences of ableism directed at disabled persons is the psychosocial process known as *deindividuation*.[2] Among people who study disability, the term refers to situations where nondisabled observers view a given disabled person as being the same as all others who share their physical, cognitive, emotional, or intellectual disability. Such objectification is frequent when labels are used to refer to people and their conditions, which often happens in clinical or medical settings. Sadly, it is not uncommon to hear a doctor or nurse refer to a patient as "the tetraplegic in ICU" or the "diabetic waiting in the ER" instead of saying the individual with tetraplegia or diabetes or a similar formulation (Dunn & Andrews, 2015).

Wright (1991) argued that such *labeling* necessarily created two outcomes representative of deindividuation linked to disability. First, placing people into categories and then labeling them (e.g., diabetics, amputees, stroke patients) is deindividuating because they are no longer seen as individuals or as distinct from one another (e.g., Wilder, 1986). Second, this labeling process suggests that there are clear distinctions among the observers (the perceivers, including medical personnel) but not those being perceived, whose identities are ignored in favor of the arbitrary disability group they find themselves in. One final ableist angle here is this one: Casual observers tend

2. In mainstream social psychology, the term "deindividuation" refers to situations where people experience a loss of perceived individuality and personal responsibility (Diener et al., 1976; Festinger et al., 1952). Such decreases in self-awareness can lead affected individuals to adopt an available group norm, which can be positive or negative (Postmes & Spears, 1998). When riots occur, for example, otherwise law-abiding citizens can become embroiled in the action around them, leading them to behave in a destructive and antisocial manner.

to assume anyone in each grouping (e.g., stroke patients) has a disability like that of all the other group members, which is false. There are many different types of strokes with different effects on cognition, emotion, and mobility, among other processes. The same holds true for other disabilities and chronic illnesses; individuation and identity are lost in favor of convenience and presumed similarity. In some ways, it is easier to deal with people in monolithic terms than as individuals with particular qualities, which of course, is a mark of prejudiced thinking and discriminatory behavior (recall Chapter 1; see also Dunn, 2015).

Thus far in this chapter, we have focused on interpreting behavior as resulting from both the person and the situation, as well as how the two interact. We also need to consider how constructive alterations of the environment can benefit people with disabilities as well as the general public.

Changing the Environment: On the Importance of Universal Design

How can the built environment be changed to aid people with disabilities? Can the first foundational principle, that of the person-environment relation, inform what sort of favorable changes can be introduced to make physical, as well as social and psychological, environments more navigable? The appropriate term for making changes to these situations is "universal design." Universal design promotes efforts to create physical, socio-recreational, work, and learning environments that can be used by a wide range of individuals and despite any disability or issues tied to age or size (e.g., Hendren, 2020; Steinfeld & Maisel, 2012; Story et al., 1998; cf. Norman, 2013). Disability scholars have been very interested in both design matters and political issues tied to universal design (e.g., Hamraie, 2017).

While they are helpful to people with disabilities, particularly where combatting ableism is tied to accessibility issues (Powell, 2013), universal design principles also benefit other individuals and groups. Curb cuts were mentioned earlier in this chapter as being beneficial for wheelchair users (indeed, they also help people who use walkers, powerchairs, and canes, among other assistive devices) as well as nondisabled people (e.g., people riding bikes or scooters, pushing strollers, using skateboards). Of course, universal design has a broader appeal than just the built world. It also applies to the creation of myriad consumer products that can be used by all people without the need for additional adaptation (e.g., automatic doors, levers, handheld and adjustable showerheads).

The late Ronald Mace (1942–1998), an architect and disability activist, coined the term "universal design" and, with colleagues affiliated with North Carolina State University, developed the seven principles of universal design. As shown in Table 3.2,

TABLE 3.2

The Seven Principles of Universal Design

1. Equitable use

The design is useful and marketable to people with diverse abilities.

These guidelines underlie principle 1:

- 1a. Provide the same means of use for all users: identical whenever possible; equivalent when not.
- 1b. Avoid segregating or stigmatizing any users.
- 1c. Provisions for privacy, security, and safety should be equally available to all users.
- 1d. Make the design appealing to all users.

2. Flexibility in use

The design accommodates a wide range of individual preferences and abilities.

These guidelines underlie principle 2:

- 2a. Provide choice in methods of use.
- 2b. Accommodate right- or left-handed access and use.
- 2c. Facilitate the user's accuracy and precision.
- 2d. Provide adaptability to the user's pace.

3. Simple and intuitive use

Use of the design is easy to understand, regardless of the user's experience, knowledge, language skills, or current concentration level.

These guidelines underlie principle 3:

- 3a. Eliminate unnecessary complexity.
- 3b. Be consistent with user expectations and intuition.
- 3c. Accommodate a wide range of literacy and language skills.
- 3d. Arrange information consistent with its importance.
- 3e. Provide effective prompting and feedback during and after task completion.

4. Perceptible information

The design communicates necessary information effectively to the user, regardless of ambient conditions or the user's sensory abilities.

These guidelines underlie principle 4:

- 4a. Use different modes (pictorial, verbal, tactile) for redundant presentation of essential information.

Continued

TABLE 3.2 *Continued*

- 4b. Provide adequate contrast between essential information and its surroundings.
- 4c. Maximize the "legibility" of essential information.
- 4d. Differentiate elements in ways that can be described (i.e., make it easy to give instructions or directions).
- 4e. Provide compatibility with a variety of techniques or devices used by people with sensory limitations.

5. Tolerance for error

The design minimizes hazards and the adverse consequences of accidental or unintended actions.

These guidelines underlie principle 5:

- 5a. Arrange elements to minimize hazards and errors: most-used elements are most accessible; hazardous elements eliminated, isolated, or shielded.
- 5b. Provide warnings about hazards and errors.
- 5c. Provide fail safe features.
- 5d. Discourage unconscious action in tasks that require vigilance.

6. Low physical effort

The design can be used efficiently and comfortably and with a minimum of fatigue.

These guidelines underlie principle 6:

- 6a. Allow user to maintain a neutral body position.
- 6b. Use reasonable operating forces.
- 6c. Minimize repetitive actions.
- 6d. Minimize sustained physical effort.

7. Size and space for approach and use

Appropriate size and space are provided for approach, reach, manipulation, and use regardless of the user's body size, posture, or mobility.

These guidelines underlie principle 7:

- 7a. Provide a clear line of sight to important elements for any seated or standing user.
- 7b. Make reach to all components comfortable for any seated or standing user.

TABLE 3.2 *Continued*

• 7c. Accommodate variations in hand and grip size. • 7d. Provide adequate space for the use of assistive devices or personal assistance.

Source: Adapted from "Defining Universal Design/The Principles of Universal Design," version 2.0 (April 1 1997) Center for Universal Design North Carolina State University (https://disabilityandmultimodality.wordpress.ncsu.edu/universal-design-ud/) and the Centre for Excellence in Universal Design Dublin Ireland (https://universaldesign.ie/about-universal-design/the-7-principles)

each principle is accompanied by a set of guidelines that provide additional depth and detail. Mace, who was disabled, was originally interested in promoting accessible housing via universal design and was an advocate for appropriate building codes and standards in the United States. The principles continue to be applied in architectural, technological, and educational settings. In addition, they also have been used to advance pedagogy where teaching writing and composition are concerned (e.g., Nielsen, 2013). Note that Mace did not claim that universal design was ever completely achievable or even an ideal solution for all situations. Rather, he believed it was more of an aspirational goal aimed at enhancing daily living within the inevitable constraints imposed by cost and affordability (Hamraie, 2017).

Of course, instances of universal design existed long before it was named and codified by Mace and the seven principles. Many architects and designers had already created spaces or objects that removed barriers to their use. Given the importance of accessibility, let's consider an example from modern architecture. The American architect Frank Lloyd Wright designed the Guggenheim Museum in New York City, which opened in 1959, intuitively using ideas that later became explicit in discussions of universal design. Still, the museum is an early example of high-quality universal design in action. The museum's interior contains a continuous spiral ramp running from the top level down to the lobby (see Figure 3.1). Wright assumed visitors would take an elevator to the top and then gradually walk down the ramp, looking at the art that was installed on the walls all along the way (of course, it is possible to walk up the ramp to the top of the museum, as well). The lore in architectural history is that Wright was not enamored of museums that required too much effort to visit and to then navigate their collections (Pfeiffer, 1991; Steinfeld & Maisel, 2012). The Guggenheim requires few or no stairs. How many other museums can make such claims? Many seem predicated on steep stairways and endless galleries connecting to yet more galleries.

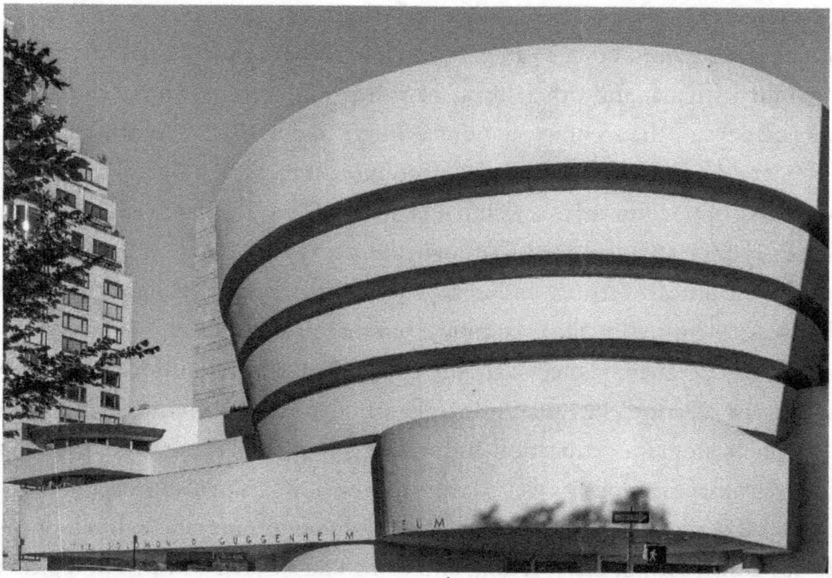

FIGURE 3.1 Frank Lloyd Wright's Guggenheim Museum, an early example of universal design, contains a continuous spiral ramp running from the top of the building down to the lobby area

Earlier, in 1949, Wright designed the Kenneth and Phyllis Laurent House, in Rockford, Illinois, a much simpler but equally elegant example of universal design. The couple wrote to Wright, asking him to design a floorplan that would afford Mr. Laurent free movement and comfort throughout the home, as he used a wheelchair (a surgery following diagnosis of a spinal tumor led to his paralysis). The result is the only Wright design focused on accommodating an owner who used a wheelchair.

The house is on one level and comprises two arcs: One contains the indoor living area, which includes an open and expansive living room, as well as a kitchen, bedrooms, and a bathroom (Pfeiffer, 2009). The bathroom was made intentionally spacious due to the owner's disability. The second arc constitutes an accessible outdoor terrace, pond, and garden, which are always in view from the living room. Ahead of its time, like the Guggenheim Museum, the home provided Mr. Laurent free movement as well as built-in, adapted furnishings (e.g., tables, a dining table, counters designed to be an appropriate height for his wheelchair to fit, and a desk in a study area) and doorways designed to accommodate the width of his wheelchair. Indeed, he credited Wright's design with granting him a long and healthy life. Like the Guggenheim Museum, the Laurent House is open to the public.

Universal design is also an important component for psychology. The American Psychological Association (APA) passed a resolution in support of universal design and accessibility in education, training, and practice (APA, 2019). The resolution details aspects of universal design that make built environments, as well as various products and services, open to all people while reducing attitudinal barriers linked to disability, stigma, and other forms of marginalization. Universal design is also important because the accommodations already provided by the Americans with Disabilities Act do not and cannot cover all architectural, sociopolitical, or attitudinal needs tied to opportunities to seek higher education (e.g., Andrews et al., 2013; Lund et al., 2014) or meaningful participation in the workforce. Universal design is also important in healthcare settings and in psychological practice settings because people with diverse identities or those coming from marginalized groups are routinely underserved (e.g., Hanass-Hancock & Alli, 2015). The APA resolution concludes with an action list meant to integrate principles of universal design into all professional development programs, education and training events, APA-sponsored workshops, and professional meetings, as well as the organization's annual convention.

Universal design considerations have also been important where developing standards for constructing, interpreting, and using educational and psychological tests is concerned (AERA, APA, & NCME, 2014). Why are such standards so critical? Tests created with universal design parameters rely on carefully defined constructs and thoughtfully chosen content, assignments, methods of response, and test procedures so that test takers' factors, such as physical or sensory impairments, do not adversely affect the use of or validity tied to a given assessment. It is still the responsibility of any psychologist who administers any psychological assessments to disabled individuals to be fair and unbiased throughout the testing and interpretation phases (for additional discussion of assessment procedures and related issues, see Andrews, 2020).

The Person and the Environment Revisited

> Every psychological event depends upon the state of the person and at the same time on the environment, although their relative importance is different in different cases.
>
> —Kurt Lewin, *Principles of Topological Psychology* (2014, p. 24)

Clinical objectivity, then, remains a key concern where universal design and psychological practice intersect in the person-environment relation. Clarity and objectivity are also called for when rehabilitation psychologists evaluate the potential role of personal factors and environmental factors in understanding the quality of a given client's person-environment relation and how particular changes or even an intervention could improve the desired outcome.

Precis and Prospects

This chapter introduced the person-environment relation, a key contribution of psychologist Kurt Lewin that shaped theorizing in both social psychology and rehabilitation psychology. Lewin argued that behavior does not originate within the person per se but, rather, through the ways the person and the perceived environment influence one another. Rehabilitation psychologists, whether practitioners or researchers, should attend to both the personal factors that affect clients and the environmental factors that impinge upon them. One challenge for perceivers is that behavior is often attributed to the person via the so-called fundamental attribution error. In turn, the psychological construct known as naive realism suggests that no one's assessment of a given situation is objective. Where disability is concerned, any negative perception on the part of an observer can trigger the fundamental negative bias. The labels people use to define others, whether casually or professionally, can adversely influence social perception, leading to deindividuation. The end of the chapter introduced universal design, where built environments and the objects in them can be created for use by all people, regardless of disability, health status, age, or size. In Chapter 4, we will move from an environmental perspective to one focused on the perspectives of disabled people themselves, the so-called insider-outsider distinction.

THOUGHT QUESTIONS

1. What is the person-environment relation? Why is it important enough to be a foundational principle for rehabilitation psychology?
2. Why are personal factors alone insufficient to explain people's behavior? Why do situational factors matter? Why is the nature of the interaction between these two factors important? How do these factors relate to understanding disability and the experience of disability?
3. Define and explain the *actor/observer bias*. How is this bias related to the *fundamental attribution error*? How can both biases be applied to disabled persons and with what consequences?
4. What is *naive realism*, and why is it a problem for perceivers, whether disability is involved or not? Late in his career, Ross suggested that naive realism is the truly fundamental attribution error. What did he mean?
5. What is the *fundamental negative bias*? Why does it appear to be an automatic, even uncontrolled, response to disability? What is *labeling*, and why is it a problem for disabled persons?

6. What is *universal design*, and why is it important for disabled individuals and other marginalized groups? What are the seven principles of universal design?
7. Why should psychologists, including rehabilitation psychologists, pay attention to issues of universal design?

4 Principle 2

THE INSIDER-OUTSIDER DISTINCTION

Foundational Principle 2: The Insider-Outsider Distinction

People with disabilities (insiders) know what life with a chronic condition is like (e.g., sometimes challenging but usually manageable), whereas casual observers (outsiders) who lack relevant experience presume that disability is defining, all encompassing, and decidedly negative.

> The role of the outsider is that of an observer, and the role of the insider is that of a participant . . . because the observer is an outsider, the impact of the situation affects him little.
>
> —Tamara Dembo (1964, p. 231)

The second foundational principle is known as the *insider-outsider distinction*, a psychosocial construct that is related to actor-observer bias, which was introduced in Chapter 3. Tamara Dembo (1902–1993), a student of Lewin and a colleague of Beatrice Wright, believed that point of view is a powerful social psychological element affecting people with disabilities and the casual nondisabled observers who become interested in them. Dembo suggested that disabled individuals (so-called insiders) know what life with a disability or other chronic condition is like (e.g., sometimes challenging but usually manageable), whereas casual observers (so-called

On the Foundational Principles of Rehabilitation Psychology. Dana S. Dunn, Oxford University Press.
 DOI: 10.1093/9780197785188.003.0004

outsiders) who lack relevant experience presume that any disability or health problem is monolithic, all encompassing, and decidedly negative (Dembo, 1964, 1970, 1982).

Similarly, disabled individuals who receive rehabilitation therapy are also insiders, as they know what such therapeutic experiences are like, whereas nondisabled outsiders can only imagine or even project their expectations onto what happens during such healthcare regimens (see also Shontz, 1982; Wright, 1989, 1991). In fact, insiders who undergo rehabilitation or other medical treatments typically enjoy a more positive outlook about their experiences than do outsiders observing the proceedings (Hamera & Shontz, 1978; Mason & Muhlenkamp, 1976). The outsiders indirectly assume that the treatment must be uncomfortable or worse, while the insiders have direct experience that the procedures in question are simply not that bad.

One reason that the insider-outsider distinction matters is because outsiders often assume that insiders are miserable due to their disability or health condition. As we will see later, such outsider catastrophizing is relatively common (recall from Chapter 3 the friend of the parent with a paralyzed adult son who perseverated about his loss of mobility), though most disabled people report reasonable levels of well-being and happiness. Not surprisingly, outsiders tend to adopt the perspective of naive realism (see Chapter 3) when viewing the lives of insiders, presuming that their own view of the reality of disability must be the correct one.

The late lawyer, disability rights activist, and author Harriet McBryde Johnson (1957–2008) shared the sorts of comments outsiders in her beloved hometown of Charleston, South Carolina, would direct at her due to her disability. In a *New York Times Magazine* article (McBryde Johnson, 2003, p. 53), she explained,

> Where I live, . . . some people call me Good Luck Lady: they consider it propitious to cross my path when a hurricane is coming and to kiss my head just before voting day. But most of the reactions are decidedly negative. Strangers on the street are moved to comment:
>
> I admire you for being out; most people would give up.
> God bless you! I'll pray for you.
> You don't let the pain hold you back, do you?
> If I had to live like you, I think I'd kill myself.

Nonetheless, she was a happy and productive person, one who especially enjoyed zooming about her city in a powered wheelchair (for her autobiography, see McBryde Johnson, 2005). But her use of that powerchair was sufficient to elicit observers' expressions of pity or the conviction that she "must" be suffering all the time.

Of course, neither the presence of a disability nor its absence is a reliable predictor of a person's quality of life. Quality of life comprises many different sources or factors within a given person, including mental health, relative level of experienced stress, physical condition, and so on (Duggan & Dijkers, 2001). As we will learn in Chapter 5, many people adjust to life with a disability with rehabilitation therapy, experience, and the passage of time. And where insiders are concerned, most are likely to regard disability as but one facet of their lives, especially if their disability is congenital (i.e., it is "all they know") or they have lived with it for some meaningful period. Or, as a disabled colleague of mine observed, "Disability is our normal" (Erin E. Andrews, personal communication, August 12, 2013).

Still, disability is but one quality among many that the insiders possess, and they may not think about it much unless they are asked about it or if some situation renders it suddenly salient (e.g., the lack of an elevator in a historic structure). Please know that this line of reasoning is not meant to downplay or, worse, to trivialize disability; rather, it is the case that no personal characteristic, whether it is physical, psychological, or dispositional, receives constant focus from the person who has it. (We rarely reflect on the color of our eyes, for example, unless we are asked to indicate it on a form or if someone complements us on it.) Thus, we should assume that insiders prefer to think about what they can accomplish; generally, they are not unduly focused on their disabilities. Indeed, insiders live with them on an ongoing basis, whereas any disability may be seen as a novelty to outsiders. What the latter miss is that they see disability as if it were an acute state ("becoming disabled") when it is a chronic but known condition that is part and parcel of the insiders' lives ("being disabled"; e.g., Kahneman, 2000).

Another subtle and important aspect of the insider-outsider distinction should not escape notice: The fact is that insiders are in the same perceptual position as outsiders where the disability experience of other insiders is concerned. Put another way, an individual with fibromyalgia can only describe their pain, fatigue, and tiredness as they experience such symptoms; they cannot characterize the disability experience or the symptomatology of anyone else who has fibromyalgia. Expecting an insider to do so—to generalize about their experience to all other insiders with a similar disability—is like asking one LGBTQ+ college student to summarize the experience of *all* LGBTQ+ college students; it is neither possible nor fair to do so (e.g., Dunn & Hammer, 2014). But this does raise an important question: Can we broaden nondisabled people's understanding of the experience of others, notably those insiders with disabilities?

Broadening People's Understanding of Disability: The Mine/Thine Exercise

Wright (1975, 1983; Wright & Lopez, 2009) described an exercise, dubbed the *mine/thine problem*, to enhance sensitivity to the actual nature of disabilities via the divergent perspectives of insiders and outsiders (i.e., foundational principle 2). At the same time, the exercise can also help people to recognize—if only for a short time—the influence of the person-environment relation (i.e., foundational principle 1) on their behavior. During the exercise, nondisabled people adopt the perspective of and act as *both* insider and outsider. For the exercise to work, participants must accept and share one or more personal qualities that could be construed as a physical, mental, emotional, or other type of "disability" or self-perceived limitation.

Wright originally conducted the exercise with college students and with medical and rehabilitation professionals. To begin, the convener defines the term "disability" for the group, who are also reminded that "everyone is handicapped [by the environment] in some way" (Wright, 1983, p. 48). Participants are then asked to jot down a disability, personal impairment, or perceived limitation on a sheet of paper. The papers are then collected, and ad hoc pairs of disabilities are created and shared with the group (either written on a blackboard or projected onto a screen at the front of the room). The convener instructs the group to locate the first pair containing their own disability and to then write the pair on a second sheet of paper. Participants then identify their own disability by underlining it. For the final step, the convener asks them to indicate their imagined choice: *"If it were possible, would you prefer to keep your own disability or the one with which it was randomly paired?"* Group members then put a star by their choice in the disability pair. The second sheets are then collected by the convener, who tallies the results. Wright (1983) reported that virtually all participants across a variety of samples (ranging between 62% and 95%) routinely decide to retain their own disability—in other words, they reject "thine" in favor of "mine."

Why bother to hold onto an identified disability in an exercise of imagination like this? Arguably, for a convincing reason: When asked to choose whether to keep or reject their disability, they are at that moment acting as both insider and outsider with respect to it. Wright (1975) presumably chose the word "problem" to describe the exercise because it triggers an interesting psychosocial conflict—either to retain a known condition or to accept an imagined and unknown one held by someone else. It follows that the disability we already know—whatever it is like—is not generally felt as disruptive to our well-being (i.e., we already live with it), as might not be the case with the one (or ones) we do not know. By holding onto their own disabilities, participants in the exercise are admitting that they do not know or really understand how other individuals live with their (unfamiliar and unknown) states. Our own disabilities are not only well-known, but they also provide some sense of comfort and perhaps contribute to our individual identities, including those tied to a disability (an issue we will explore in Chapter 5). Unknown or unfamiliar conditions are challenging because they represent uncertainty and possibly threat.

Wright (1983) provided a variety of psychosocial explanations for why retaining a known disability in the mine/thine problem might seem to be a reasonable decision. Table 4.1 lists and defines some of these explanations. One explanation—perhaps *familiarity*—may be sufficient to cover a given individual's motivation to retain their own disability. However, another individual might appeal to several of the explanations listed in Table 4.1 simultaneously. Which one or ones people choose is arguably less important than recognizing the consistency with which participants in the exercise hold onto their self-reported disabilities.

Beyond a Sensitizing Exercise: Changing Minds, Changing Attitudes

Although it may have been used as a sensitizing exercise in some educational and rehabilitation settings, there are not many publications on the mine/thine problem. Dunn, Fisher, and Beard (2012) decided to conduct two studies using the basic problem design: one conceptual replication and an extension study. The goal was to determine if current groups of students, professionals, and adults still respond to the task as they did in Wright's samples. Following the usual procedure, the replication study recruited 52 participants and found that 78% of them chose to retain their own disability. When asked to explain why they preferred their own disabilities, many respondents conveyed concern about navigating their daily situations with an unfamiliar disability (essentially recalling many of the explanations summarized in Table 4.1).

In contrast, the extension study had two additional goals. First, Dunn et al. (2012) wanted to demonstrate that retaining a disability was not due to the perceived severity of the paired (unfamiliar) disability but was a genuine choice. To do so, a separate sample of 96 people rated a list of disabilities on a 9-point scale of severity (where higher scores indicated a perception of greater severity). During the exercise, half of the participants were assigned a disability that was rated as less severe than their own, while the other half received one that was rated as more severe than their disability. For instance, blindness ($M = 8.01$) was rated as more severe than stuttering ($M = 3.28$) or colorblindness ($M = 2.34$).

TABLE 4.1

Possible Explanations for Why Mine/Thine Problem Participants Retain Their Own Disabilities

Familiarity: A known disability puts people at ease. The consistent results from the mine/thine problem imply that changing a familiar aspect of oneself is a challenge, even when it is only imagined.

Self-identity: If a disability has always been there, living without it is difficult to do. Besides being a familiar quality, a disability can represent an important part of oneself, one's identity, and personal history (e.g., Dunn & Burcaw, 2013).

Positive aspects or secondary gains: Some individuals want to keep a disability because they believe it affords them particular advantages (so-called secondary gains). Associating a positive quality with a disability or chronic health condition could represent a form of benefit finding (e.g., slowing down daily routines, focusing on what matters in daily life), as well as cognitive adaptation (e.g., Tennen & Affleck, 2002). However, being excused from a duty or responsibility is not a positive aspect or a secondary gain.

Coping: Knowing how to live day to day with a disability or health condition is beneficial; adapting to a new condition triggers uncertainty, perhaps leading to the desire to retain one's own disability.

Reactance: Psychological reactance happens when people believe they are being induced to give up something of value (like a positive aspect or a secondary gain), especially their behavioral freedom (i.e., giving up a known disability for an unknown one) (Brehm & Brehm, 1981).

Energy-conservation motives: Despite the fact that the exercise involves an imaginary situation, participants might still expect that changes tied to accepting a novel disability could be disruptive and taxing where daily living is concerned. Exchanging the known for the unknown could require greater use of personal energy than is desirable.

Psychological spread: Spread occurs when some negative feature (e.g., a stigma, a disability) directs subsequent negative associations that, though they are usually arbitrary, can color later social judgments. If an unknown disability is seen as worse than one's own, that negativity might "spread" and compromise other abilities (the spread effect is discussed in detail later in this chapter).

Source: Adapted from Dunn (2015); Dunn Fisher & Beard (2013); Wright (1983)

The second goal of Dunn et al.'s (2012) extension study was to learn if taking part in the exercise changed people's minds about disability so that their beliefs became more positive immediately after completing the study and lasted two weeks beyond that point. To do so, all participants completed the Scale of Attitudes Towards Disabled Persons (SADP) at three times: one-week before the exercise, immediately following the exercise, and two weeks after the exercise. The SADP comprises 24 items designed to assess an individual's attitudes toward people with disabilities as a group (higher scores on the measure indicate more favorable attitudes; Antonak, 1981; Antonak & Livneh, 1988).

The results indicated that disability severity (whether more or less) had little effect on the participants' decisions, as 90% of them preferred to retain their own disability. Where attitudes were concerned, participants were more favorably (and significantly) disposed toward disabled people as a group immediately after the exercise (M = 117.10) and two weeks later (M = 119.22) compared to the preexercise assessment (M = 110.41). Wright's intuition was correct: Not only does the exercise sensitize people to the insider-outsider distinction, but it also actually leads to more positive attitudes toward disability and disabled people immediately afterward and for at least two subsequent weeks.

We now turn to halo effects, what is known as inspiration porn, and spread.

Halo Effects, Inspiration Porn, and Spread Effects

The social psychologist Solomon Asch (1946) convincingly demonstrated that the presence of one personality trait usually leads perceivers to anticipate the presence of other, similar traits. The original experiment was quite simple: One group of participants heard about a person who was described as "intelligent, skillful, industrious, warm, determined, practical, cautious." Another group heard the same list with one exception—the word "cold" was substituted for the word "warm." Would such a subtle change matter? Quite a bit, as the two groups formed very different impressions of the target person. The "warm" group imagined the person as being more generous, funny, happy, and good-natured than did the "cold" group. Asch theorized that such perceptual differences happen because warm and cold are central traits that decidedly influence perceivers to infer the presence (or absence, for that matter) of other related traits, thereby affecting the gist of their overall impressions (see also Kelley, 1950; Stapel & Kooman, 2000).

When people's judgments of another person are positive, psychologists label the event a *halo effect.* In other words, one favorable quality leads perceivers to assume other ones are also present—as if the individual possessed a halo above their head, signifying their inherent goodness or even "saintliness." One well-known example from social psychology is the "what is beautiful is good" stereotype (Dion et al., 1972), where an attractive person is presumed to also be happy, intelligent, successful, confident, assertive, well-adjusted—and often vain (Eagly et al., 1991). Like any functional stereotype, halo effects promote quick thinking that leads to an in-the-moment judgment about another person. Besides saving time and cognitive effort, halo effects allow perceivers to proceed with feelings of certainty about the target person (e.g., Fiske & Taylor, 2021).

Can the presence of a disability trigger a halo effect? Most certainly. Sometimes a halo effect linked to a disabled person allows the outsider to "see" some beneficent qualities attached to the insider, such as cheerfulness, politeness, and even happiness, and these can compensate for the negative aspects associated with disability. Yet being seen as having such "unreal goodness" can be socially off-putting to the insider and even annoying, as it may cause the observer to act in some overly solicitous ways. Such halo effects are especially likely to befall children with disabilities, who may be viewed as in need of protection due to their presumed (if unproven or demonstrated) fragility (Dunn, 2015). These sorts of halo effects have been dubbed the "kindness norm," which means that outsiders should "be kind to the less fortunate" (Kleck, 1968), another form of objectification and ableism.

INSPIRATION PORN?

Sometimes halo effects tied to a disabled person can become even more pronounced, so that the person is admired and even sensationalized for living with a disability (after his horse-riding accident, the late actor Christopher Reeve, who pledged to walk again, exemplified this social role—and not without controversy; see, for example, McBryde Johnson, 2005). Disability culture labels such cases *inspiration porn* (Grue, 2016). Examples abound on social media and often employ a "feel good" moment, as when a disabled child is "adopted" by an athletic team as a mascot or honorary "coach," one who might get to shoot hoops with the basketball players during a warmup before a game; if the disabled child makes a basket, so much the better! Alternatively, disabled people going about their normal business can sometimes be applauded for doing normal activities of living—like driving, shopping in a grocery store for themselves, having a hobby, or even raising a family. A common element is that nondisabled outsiders put the person on a metaphorical pedestal and praise them for doing things that seem difficult due to the presence of their disability but that would not receive undue or even any recognition if they were performed by a nondisabled person. As Serlin (2015) observed, these sorts of images can be sentimental or used for quasi-motivational purposes that "have the dual function of making the nondisabled feel better about themselves while simultaneously holding the average disabled person to an impossibly high standard" (p. 43).

The late Australian comedian and disability activist Stella Young, who likely coined the term "inspiration porn," noted that such images usually show disabled individuals doing mundane things, such as running, playing, drawing, or taking part in a sport. These portrayals are then used to urge on nondisabled viewers with "bumper sticker" philosophies like "just do it," "quit making excuses," "can't means won't," or "if they can, you can." Inspiration porn is not about insiders, nor is it created for them; its goal is to inspire outsiders—which means it is yet another objectifying form of ableism (recall Chapter 1).

If disabled persons complain about the exploitative nature of these memes or other representations, they risk being metaphorically pushed off their pedestals by outsiders for being bitter and ungrateful and for refusing to play their assigned social roles (Young, 2012). In other words, insiders risk earning a negative halo from outsiders.

NEGATIVE HALO EFFECTS OR SPREAD

Negative halo effects exist, of course, though in rehabilitation psychology and the social psychology of disability, they are usually called *spread effects* (Dembo et al., 1956; Wright, 1964, 1983) or simply *spread* (spread was introduced and defined at the bottom of Table 4.1 as a possible reason participants choose to retain their own disability in the mine/thine exercise). Spread occurs when an outsider encounters an insider and responds to some disability cue—slow or slurred speech, a stutter, an atypical gait when walking, use of a cane or a wheelchair, a missing limb or limbs, presence of an aid or a service animal, and so on—that elicits expectations that other qualities, presumed to be negatively valanced, are also present (i.e., bad is stronger than good; recall Chapter 3). Perhaps normative social perception would acknowledge the presence of a disability by focusing on a single cue but not hypothesizing that other negative qualities are also there. Unfortunately, that is not how spread works; instead, it taints other abilities or even neutral qualities and turns them into disabilities, or a form of collateral damage. Slow or slurred speech *must* mean that the insider's intelligence or memory is linked to their vocalizations, or that personal aid or trained dog points to the insider's inherent helplessness at navigating about alone.

An accompanying problem occurs when the insider suspects that they are the target of spread-based expectations, so that the outsider (or outsiders) is socially devaluing them. This can happen in subtle ways (e.g., limited eye contact, too much social distance, awkward chitchat) or in more direct ones (e.g., speaking to the aid and not the insider about the latter, talking in a loud, slow voice or perhaps in a baby-talk like manner; see, for example, Gouvier et al., 1994; Liesener & Mills, 1999). The point is that what might have been a cordial or even friendly, productive, and meaningful social encounter is lost, so that poor-quality communication and the automatic exchange of confirmed stereotypes on both sides occur (e.g., Snyder et al., 1977). Wright (1983) also observed that spread effects happen when other intersectional factors are present, such as race, sex, ethnicity, religion, or nationality; we might also add sexual orientation and social class, among other possibilities (recall Chapter 2).

Stereotyping Disabilities

Whether disabled or not, halo and spread effects are tied to the perception of persons. Person perception often entails categorizing people (recall Chapter 1), with the consequence that stereotypes are invoked that reduce or eliminate concern for individuality and identity. Fiske (2011) suggested that the stereotyping of various social groups, including disabled individuals, occurs when they are evaluated on two important dimensions of judgment: *warmth* and *competence*. Each of these dimensions has two poles that elicit distinct emotional reactions. People who trigger warmth are seen as friendly and worthy of trust, while those deemed cold (i.e., low warmth) are thought of as adversaries or exploiters. Competent individuals habitually are imbued with a high status, while low-status people are seen as incompetent or ineffectual.

The resulting four combinations are quick guides for viewing social groups in emotional terms (Fiske, 2011; Fiske et al., 2002; see also, Cuddy et al., 2007, 2008; Dovidio et al., 2011; see also, Wu & Fiske, 2019). To perceivers, those judged as high in warmth and competence are deemed allies or members of one's own ingroup (e.g., middle-class individuals, fellow Americans). However, groups that attract warm feelings but are also deemed to be incompetent—like disabled persons and older adults—prompt an ambivalent mix of feelings, generally pity and sympathy. Low-warmth but high-competence groups include wealthy people, professionals, Asians and people of Asian descent, and Jews, all of whom are subject to perceivers' envy. Finally, groups perceived to be low on both warmth and competence (e.g., people who use drugs, those experiencing homelessness, or those with low incomes) generate feelings of disgust, resentment, and sometimes even anger.

Our analysis of the insider-outsider distinction reveals consequences for outsider perception of insiders as individuals or as the member of some larger group. How can outsiders become aware that the actual lived experience of insiders differs from their expectations tied to disability? Just as observers in the actor/observer bias situation should learn to become attuned to environmental influences and constraints on behavior, outsiders in the insider-outsider distinction need to listen and to learn to accept the veracity of insider experiences, especially when the claim is that disability "while never wished for—may simply not be as wholly disastrous as imagined" (Fine & Asch, 1988, p. 11).

Accepting Insider Perspectives as Genuine

A main challenge of promoting insider perspectives is finding meaningful ways to share them with outsiders. Clearly, clinical as well as educational contexts are implicated here, and rehabilitation training occurs in both. An important part of that training should be explaining the inherent perceptual biases present in the insider-outsider distinction and helping students and interns, as well as seasoned professionals and other medical staff, to recognize them.

A second challenge tied to elucidating insider perspectives is doing so in a way that does not trivialize the experience of disability or veer off into testimonials that are like inspiration porn. This effort requires identifying individuating exemplars and then helping rehabilitation professionals and students to find their own exemplars in their work with clients. Note that this does not mean that all clients necessarily will have positive insider experiences to share; the rehabilitation psychology literature is replete with research highlighting various psychosocial problems and comorbidities tied to the onset or consequences of disability. As we will learn in Chapter 5, not all clients adjust to disabling experiences in the same way or on similar timelines.

Nonetheless, the two examples reviewed here are meant to be a starting point for adopting the perspective of the insider; readers should try to collect their own examples through their reading, practice work, teaching, or research. Other examples may be found in Chapter 5, which discusses disability identity issues (see, for example, Dunn & Burcaw, 2013, for other exemplar candidates).

MARK ZUPAN

During part of his college career, Mark Zupan, was a member of a university soccer team.[1] After a game, he and some teammates celebrated their success at a college bar. After downing many free drinks, Zupan left the bar at midnight and decided to

1. I am grateful to Thomas Gilovich and the late Lee Ross, authors of *The Wisest One in the Room*, where I learned of Mark Zupan's story.

sleep off his bender in the bed of a teammate's pickup truck. The teammate also got drunk, left the bar two hours later, and thought he could safely drive the two miles back to his dorm. He could not: Taking an exit ramp too fast, he lost control of the vehicle, crashing into a fence and having no clue that Zupan was asleep in the truck bed. The accident's force threw Zupan from the back of the truck and into a nearby drainage canal. Zupan recalls not being able to feel anything in his legs after that. His teammate was quickly arrested for driving under the influence (DUI), and the truck was towed away. No one knew Zupan was in the ditch, holding onto a tree branch to keep his head above the briny water. Discovered the next day, he was hospitalized and learned that his injured spine was irreparable. He was eventually diagnosed with what is known as incomplete quadriplegia, which means he still retained some function and feeling in his arms and legs.[2]

What sort of psychological toll did this take on Zupan? Now that you have read about outsider perspectives, you can imagine how the paragraph you just read might be parsed by some: Who would not become depressed or withdrawn after such an event? Would he or anyone in a similar circumstance ever describe themselves as happy or satisfied again? Well, Zupan returned to athletics, becoming a champion wheelchair rugby player as well as once more a happy person.[3] Reflecting on the accident in his book, *Gimp* (Zupan, 2006), he wrote,

> In truth, my accident has been the best thing that could have ever happened to me. I'm not trying to be glib when I say this, or rationalize my mistakes, or offer a steaming bowl of bullshit-flavored Chicken Soup for the Soul. What I am saying is that it has been the single most defining event of my life. And without it, I wouldn't have seen the things I've seen, done the things I've done and met so many incredible people. I wouldn't have become a world class athlete. I wouldn't have come to understand my friends and family the way I do, and feel the kind of love they have for me and I have for them (p. 6).

Is Zupan's experience a common one for people with spinal cord injuries? Would most outsiders anticipate that most insiders adjust to their disabilities across time? We know from Harriet McBryde Johnson's (2003) encounters with the public presented earlier in this chapter that many people she meets claim they "would give up" or say things like "If I had to live like you, I think I'd kill myself." Perhaps we can imagine that some of the acquaintances and casual observers encountered

2. In Zupan's case, he was eventually able to walk short distances using crutches.
3. He is a Paralympic medal winner as well as the star of the MTV/ThinkFilm documentary *Murderball.*

in the weeks and months following the accident, if not his family and friends, felt the same way.

What research regarding the aftermath of spinal cord injury does show is that most individuals who lose the use of their limbs do lead lives with approximately the same level of happiness they experienced before their losses (as well as the same relative levels of frustration, woe, and other feelings). Indeed, a longitudinal study showed that over 85% of a sample of people who were paralyzed by spinal cord injuries reported their quality of life as *average* or *above average*—and one out of every four members of the sample described their lives as almost *ideal* (Hall et al., 1999). So, Mark Zupan's experience is not a rarity (except perhaps for his athletic prowess); like him, other people who acquire disabilities do adapt. One lesson here is that outsiders (including those who become insiders) may overestimate people's abilities (particularly their own) to forecast future feelings accurately; disability onset may be anticipated to be much worse than the actual experience turns out to be (see, for example, Wilson & Gilbert, 2003; Wilson et al., 2000; see also, Dunn, 2015, 2019d).

Yet, interestingly, but given the compelling nature of the insider-outsider distinction, not surprisingly, other research evidence finds that very few medical professionals who work with spinal cord injuries—fewer than one doctor or nurse in five—accept that their own lives would be comparably satisfying if they experienced a similar injury (Gerhart et al., 1994). These (and presumably other) medical and rehabilitation professionals forget that *being* disabled is not at all the same experience as *becoming* disabled; the former becomes a chronic but familiar state, while the latter is an acute, stressful, and perhaps even painful event (Dunn, 2015; Kahneman, 2000). As we will see in Chapter 5, adjustment to disability means that as a personal quality, one's disability becomes one of many other personal qualities; thus, it likely becomes a source of concern only occasionally, not continually (recall foundational principle 1, the person-environment relation; see Chapter 3).

Let's consider a second example of an insider perspective.

Elsie Roy and Deaf Gain

Elsie Roy is creative designer as well as a disability rights lawyer. In a well-known TED talk, she claimed, "I believe that losing my hearing was one of the greatest gifts I've ever received" (TED, 2016). Sound familiar? This comment is a variation on those made by Mark Zupan. Although hearing loss is a common disability, it is still generally viewed negatively. Consider a perspective shared by Bauman and Murry (2014): After many visits to audiologists and other doctors, a performance artist who acquired hearing loss as a child remarked, "Why had all the doctors told me I was losing my hearing, and not a single one told me I was gaining my deafness?"

Roy, too, believes that being Deaf provides her with a particular way to encounter the world and to reframe it in constructive ways that can help others. She believes her disability provides her with design insights that can solve a variety of societal problems. To that end, she believes that "when we design for disability first, you often stumble upon solutions that are better than those when we design for the norm" (TED, 2016). Her view of "design thinking" is one that is intended to shift existing mindsets into new directions so that more creative solutions emerge where accommodating disability is concerned.

This perspective and its underlying philosophy are representative of what is known as Deaf Gain, a term encompassing contributions made by Deaf individuals and the Deaf community and highlighting how deafness has led to the development of sign language and closed captioning as important forms of communication (Bauman & Murray, 2014). Adherents of Deaf Gain ask a critical question: Is the world is better off with Deaf people and their signed languages, or should the focus be on eliminating deafness, say, via cochlear implants and other biomedical interventions? Or would something be lost? Would our social world truly benefit if hearing loss were eliminated?

Elsie Roy and others believe that no, that the Deaf have improved the world for everyone—via language, art, and science, among other arenas—while adding a distinct culture to the mix (recall Chapter 2). In fact, hearing loss can be understood to represent an individual and social gain, one that stands in the way of the perils of monocultural vulnerability (i.e., seeing the absence of disability and outsiders as representative of what is "normal," thereby missing insights from various insider groups). Deaf Gain may offer unexpected opportunities for all. As Bauman and Murray (2014), professors at Gallaudet University (an institution dedicated to educating Deaf and hard of hearing students) observe,

> Deaf individuals experience a host of visual-tactile processing acuities that have the potential to provide insights into the wider practices of say, architecture, filmmaking, video game design, bilingual education[4], monitoring surveillance videos, and engaging in prolonged eye contact.

Perhaps outsiders should extend the notion of disability gain to other insiders besides the Deaf. Insiders may have much to teach, and outsiders may welcome the opportunity to learn from them.

4. https://www.psychologytoday.com/us/basics/education

Precis and Prospects

> There is no truth. There is only perception.
>
> —Gustave Flaubert (1982, p. xii)

To some degree, Flaubert was correct: Our perceptions do guide us, and sometimes their veracity is questionable. Yet, as we have learned about foundational principle 2 in this chapter, we do need to attend to and trust the perspectives of insiders when they claim that disability is not necessarily an ongoing preoccupation. For their part, outsiders must recognize that their projected expectations on what disability is like can be quite wrong, as being disabled is a different matter than becoming disabled. Use of the mine/thine exercise can help individuals see their own experience simultaneously as both insider and outsider. Retaining one's own disability is a way to perceive like an insider and to change our outsider attitudes toward disability in a more favorable direction. Halo and spread effects are on the same continuum; the former is positively valanced, the latter negatively so. Inspiration porn misleads outsiders while it objectifies insiders. When we move from perceiving the individual to the group, stereotypes tend to be used, such that resulting attitudes toward disabled people become ambivalent; they are viewed with warmth but seen as incompetent. In Chapter 5, we will explore the ways that individuals adjust to congenital and acquired disabilities, as well as the psychosocial consequences therein.

THOUGHT QUESTIONS

1. Why is the insider-outsider distinction so important? How is it related to actor/observer bias, discussed in Chapter 3?
2. Why is being disabled a different psychological proposition than becoming disabled?
3. Summarize the mine/thine exercise: How does it help outsiders to also think like insiders? Why does the level of severity of a paired disability rarely lead participants to choose the paired disability? How does taking part in the exercise seem to change people's attitudes in positive ways?
4. What are halo effects? How are they related to disability and sometimes inspiration porn?
5. What is spread or the spread effect? How is it tied to the halo effect?
6. As a group, how can disabled people be received with warmth but also viewed as incompetent? What are the consequences of such perspectives?
7. Identify some clinical implications that could be tied to the insider-outsider distinction.

5 Principle 3
ADJUSTMENT TO DISABILITY

Foundational Principle 3: Adjustment to Disability

Coping with a disability or chronic illness is an ongoing dynamic process, one that is dependent on making constructive changes to the social and physical environment.

> Acceptance in the sense of preference is certainly not unknown among people who have a disability. There are those who would not relinquish the disability even if they could. There are those who are glad they are deaf and even wish their children to be. . . . A disability can become an inextricable part of one's identity and one's life. To cast it aside can signal too basic a restructuring and a relinquishing of aspect and values that are too important.
>
> —Beatrice A. Wright (1983, p. 159)

> For there is nothing either good or bad, but that thinking makes it so.
>
> —Hamlet (Act II, Scene II)

Is there a right way to adjust and cope with disability? When does such adjustment turn into an acceptance of the disability? Do people with congenital disabilities adjust in a different manner than those who acquire a disability later in life? How do we know (indeed, can we know) when a given individual has successfully adjusted

On the Foundational Principles of Rehabilitation Psychology. Dana S. Dunn, Oxford University Press.
 DOI: 10.1093/9780197785188.003.0005

to their disability? These and related questions are asked by people with disabilities, their families and caregivers, and the rehabilitation, medical, and nursing professionals who treat or work with them. Casual observers—that is, outsiders to the experience of disability (recall Chapter 4)—may ask slightly different questions, though they, too, essentially want to know how disabled persons deal with their fates.

Psychosocial adjustment to disability is likely more of a process than a destination. Humans like the idea of closure, but it may be that for some people, adjustment to disability continues across their lives, whereas others cope with the challenge at a much faster pace. And what about individuals with congenital disabilities—do they also experience adjustment? Foundational principle 3 emphasizes that adjustment is an ongoing and dynamic process, one focusing on making constructive social and environmental changes as needed, a fact that harkens back to the person-environment relation (foundational principle 1).

Consider this example of adjustment to disability. Years ago, a close friend of mine who taught at my university had a stroke. His first few days in the hospital were difficult, and initially, he was upset and confused by his condition. As we learned in Chapter 4, *becoming disabled* can be a stressful, even traumatic set of events (e.g., Kahneman, 2000). Following a hospital stay, he was moved to an excellent rehabilitation facility, and for a few weeks, he underwent intensive rehabilitation therapy, relearning how to do activities of daily living and gradually learning to walk again. He had some aphasia, so other therapists worked on speech skills with him. When he returned home, he began to adapt to his situation, learning to navigate inside and around the house. He had hoped to eventually return to full-time teaching, but the aphasia prevented him from doing so (his speech production was slower than it was before the stroke, but he was easily understood, and his memory and other cognitive faculties were not affected; however, lecturing, running class discussions, and grading papers and exams would have been too taxing on his energy). In the end, he remained on disability leave and then took early retirement. He told me that moving out of his office made for a sad and difficult day, but the next day he told me he was "over it." In other words, he was now *being disabled*; the period of becoming disabled was over.

Afterward, he continued to visit campus daily to see me and our other friends. I recall being asked by various and sundry people, "How is he doing?" with looks of sadness and concern. I replied, "He has adjusted to his new circumstance very well." In fact, he and I laughed and gossiped about campus politics as we had always done, and his stroke was rarely a topic of discussion. I write this not to suggest that we avoided it, but rather, it was not a focus of major concern any longer; he had adapted to his situation. Within several months, he got a modified steering wheel for his car and got another form of his autonomy back. Although he could not teach in the classroom again, he was able to retain his role as an assistant coach for the college's football team, so his teaching went on in a slightly different form. As of this writing, he has moved to a local retirement community where he tends a garden of potted plants on his patio and continues to see his family and friends, like me.

Do most people who experience a stroke react this way? I suspect not, but many probably do. More broadly, why do some people respond to disability or other negative events with alacrity and resolve, while others struggle and are to some extent overcome by them? Or, as Wright (1983) put it, they "succumb." Adjusting to or coping with disability is not a "yes" or "no" proposition; both qualities are on a continuum where there may be movement both forward and backward, good days and bad ones, too. What needs to be remembered is that nondisabled outsiders invariably assume that disabled insiders will experience a lower quality of life, though research suggests otherwise (e.g., Ubel et al., 2003). Studies of individuals with colostomies (Boyd et al., 1990) and rheumatoid arthritis (Hurst et al., 1994) and those who receive dialysis (Riis et al. 2005; Sackett & Torrance, 1978) demonstrate reasonable adjustment. Like Hamlet, Prince of Denmark, how people frame their disability or chronic health-related experiences—as favorable or unfavorable, as navigable or tragic—makes quite a bit of difference to their coping and adjustment processes.

Coping with, Adapting, and Adjusting to Disability: A Brief Overview

A considerable amount of scholarly inquiry has explored how individuals adjust to acquired disabilities (see, for example, Brenner et al., 2019; Heinemann, 1995; Li & Moore, 1998; Meade et al., in press; Shontz, 1977; Smedema et al., 2009; Wright, 1983). Factors like body image, stress, self-concept, and loss and grieving influence the quality of life experienced by people who acquire disabilities and other chronic health conditions (Livneh & Antonak, 2005). Naturally, perhaps, the primary focus is on negative or maladaptive responses to disability (Kendall & Buys, 1998), which in turn can predict subsequent mental and physical health status, as well as outcomes linked to rehabilitation therapy (Livneh et al., 2004).

Yet Wright (1983) identified a variety of qualities illustrating good coping with disability. As shown in Table 5.1, these qualities can be displayed or enacted by the disabled individual or in cooperation with family members, friends, or rehabilitation professionals. The list in Table 5.1 is by no means exhaustive, and readers can likely suggest additional entries. Examples of low or poor coping can be demonstrated by considering the opposite behaviors shown in Table 5.1. The first entry could be recast as "dependent and inactive," and so on.

TABLE 5.1

Insider Qualities Associated with Effective Coping with Disability
Is independent and active
Engages and participates in social, vocational, and leisure activities
Concentrates on intrinsic qualities and perceived assets (see Chapter 6)
Does not devalue the self, skills, or limitations
Exerts effort to change or eliminate physical and psychosocial barriers
Sees any negative aspects in daily life as manageable
Accepts and understands any limits
Welcomes helpful medical procedures, assistive devices (e.g., cane, prostheses), or helpers (e.g., personal aids, service animals)

Source: Adapted from Dunn (2015, p. 79, Table 5.1) and Wright (1983, p. 195, Figure 9.1)

The use of terms like coping, adaptation, and adjustment suggest that a disabling or other chronic health state is not congenital; rather, its occurrence is linked to some acute event, such as an accident or the onset of a disease. We will discuss the differences between and consequences of acquired versus congenital disabilities later in this chapter. When a disabling event occurs, the affected individual starts a process of psychosocial adaptation, one requiring coming to terms with physical, social, and psychological changes that will gradually become part of the self, identity, and body image and the accompanying rhythms of daily living. *Adaptation* involves an active and open-ended somatopsychological (i.e., how physique affects self-image and behavior; Barker et al., 1953; Wright, 1983) process (see Chapter 7) that newly disabled people experience as they move toward an idealized objective of *adjustment* (Livneh & Antonak, 1997). Adjustment is reached when the affected person is accepting of and satisfied with their own person-environment relation (i.e., foundational principle 1, Chapter 3) so that bodily changes or physical losses no longer represent preoccupations, allowing for a focus on abilities and assets (see Chapter 6) and things that can be accomplished. Psychosocial adjustment is apparent when there is a solid link between the disabled person's perception of subjective experience and the situation in which they live (Livneh & Antonak, 1997; Roessler & Bolton, 1978). Not all people will adjust to their conditions, as adaptation will be easier for some than for others. Hallmarks of adjustment include the coping qualities noted in Table 5.1, as well as displaying active problem solving, a positive self-concept and high self-esteem, and a sense of personal mastery, among other favorable attitudes and behaviors.

BEYOND ADAPTATION AND ADJUSTMENT: ACCEPTANCE

Wright (1960, 1983) believed that the continuum from adaptation to adjustment could constructively be expanded by including the concept of acceptance of a disability. In Wright's view, the term "acceptance" is appropriately applied when a disability or other chronic condition is incorporated into the affected individual's self-concept. Acceptance occurs when the individual views their condition as a *nondevaluing* outcome (Wright's language) that does not reduce their inherent self-worth, ongoing psychosocial functioning, or a belief in future prospects. Acceptance is not being "resigned to one's fate" or attempting to "pass" by covering up a disability or mimicking the actions of nondisabled outsiders. Wright saw acceptance as a realistic response, one where the disability is recognized for what it is and what it entails, along with a continuing desire to "improve the improvable" (Wright, 1983, p. 159; see also Kerr, 1961). Acceptance means recognizing functional achievements without the burden of frequently revisiting or, worse, ruminating on what can no longer be done (Dembo et al., 1956; Wright, 1960).

MIND THE HEDONIC TREADMILL

One influence on adjustment to both good and bad events that cannot be overlooked is the so-called hedonic treadmill. Brickman et al. (1978) ran a study involving individuals with acquired spinal cord injuries (SCIs) and found that the participants reported happiness levels close to those of nondisabled individuals.[1] These findings led the researchers to propose the idea of a *hedonic treadmill*, where psychologically speaking, people's responses to both good and bad events are viewed as temporary (Brickman & Campbell, 1971; Helson, 1964). As people move through time and further away from some valanced event (e.g., a disabling accident, a financial windfall), they appear to adjust to both positive and negative outcomes, seeming to return to the original (perhaps their natural) set point of happiness (see also Lyubomirsky et al., 2005; but see Sheldon & Lyubomirsky, 2021, which is discussed in Chapter 6). Most of us can recall desired purchases—a new car, a smartphone, a new article of clothing—that made us happy at the time, yet our positive feelings gradually dissipated as the item lost its novelty and soon became one of many other possessions (e.g., Kasser, 2002). Yet where adversity is concerned, perhaps there is a beneficial side to transitory feelings: We adjust to negative events and eventually return to our

1. Brickman and colleagues' (1978) article also reported finding that across time, lottery winners tend not to be much happier than nonwinners, a result that may demonstrate the often-short-lived impact of material acquisitions; see, for example, Kasser, 2002.

previous level of well-being. Wouldn't this be an adaptive response to disability or other chronic health conditions?

The late Ed Diener (1946–2021) and his colleagues did a careful review of the classic Brickman et al. (1978) study, demonstrating that the favorable adaptation of the people with SCIs was in actuality significantly lower than that reported by the study's control group (Diener et al., 2006). Why did the mythical conclusions about hedonic adaptation persist for so long? How could so many readers and researchers alike misinterpret the results? They may have misread a table that contained the self-reported future predicted happiness of the SCI group, which was a hoped for but *future projection* and not one based on longitudinal findings tied to any return to baseline happiness (Biswas-Diener, 2013). What we can presume is that symptoms of depression, a common secondary complication linked with SCIs, likely caused the lower mean levels among the SCI group (Elliott & Kennedy, 2004). Other researchers also find that after an SCI, affected people report lower levels of relative happiness compared to the general population, and especially as a function of the severity of their acquired disability (Dijkers, 1997, 2005; Hammell, 2004; Lucas, 2007a, 2007b).

So, people do adjust and return to baseline levels of positive affect in some but not all cases. Some negative events, including a disabling event, can permanently alter individuals reported subjective well-being. As Diener and colleagues (2006) observed, "although people with paraplegia and other individuals with disabilities are not subjectively miserable, happiness levels do seem to be strongly affected by this important life circumstance" (p. 307). Thus, the hedonic treadmill metaphor may apply in some but not all situations, an important point that rehabilitation professionals should keep in mind when counseling their clients (for further discussion of these and related issues, see Dunn, 2015; Dunn et al., 2009; Smith et al., 2009).

ANOTHER INFLUENCE: POSITIVE PSYCHOLOGY

Since the advent of positive psychology in the late 1990s, many rehabilitation psychologists have become interested in ways to help their disabled clients not simply to adjust but to flourish by developing positive character strengths and building lives that have meaning and purpose. Others have examined resilient reactions to the onset of disability and other chronic illnesses (see, for example, Dunn, 2018; Dunn et al., 2013; Dunn, Uswatte, & Elliott, 2021; Ehde, 2010; Wehmeyer, 2013; Wehmeyer & Dunn, 2022b; Andrews et al., in press). In a real sense, however, the field of rehabilitation psychology has always been interested in identifying salutary factors or constructive interventions that can aid people with disabilities to lead fuller and happier lives. Interest in positive psychology has broadened the variety and scope of applications aimed at exploring the positive sides of disability. This book is not about positive psychology per se, but the foundational principles and their beneficial utility bear some relation to positive psychology. Indeed, later in this chapter, we will discuss topics that relate to positive psychology, including psychosocial resilience and finding positive meaning.

Identity Formation and Disability Identity

A key factor in promoting adjustment and coping with disability is the idea of identity formation. In other words, to what degree is a disability incorporated into a person's identity, ideally in a positive manner. Adjustment to disability is clearly related to disability identity formation, and sometimes each can be difficult to discern from the other, though they are not hypothesized to be the same process (Forber-Pratt et al., 2018). The former process emphasizes how a given individual thinks, feels, and behaves in response to either a congenital or an acquired disability, whereas the latter process involves how and whether disability is a core part of that person's sense of self.

A person with chronic pain might have adjusted to their disability, functioning well in the workplace, at home, and when socializing with friends. In all three spheres of life the individual is seen as active and successful. Yet it is possible that this person distances themselves from the disability by trying to "pass" as nondisabled (i.e., chronic pain may not be noticeable to casual observers), avoiding connections with disabled others in favor of nondisabled peers and friends and not thinking of themselves as disabled, so that the very idea is of no relevance to their personal identity or private or public life. Alternatively, of course, disability could be the center of the person's identity, as indicated by their active involvement in the local disability community as well as engagement in advocacy efforts to promote civil rights and equity issues for the disabled regionally and even nationally. And, finally, one can imagine another individual who has conflicted feelings—both pro and con—regarding their disabled status, so that they feel, act, and think about disability in an ambivalent manner. As always, people's identities can be surprisingly complex and may change depending upon the situations they encounter.

GILL'S MODEL OF DISABILITY IDENTITY DEVELOPMENT

Carol Gill, a disabled psychologist whose work on disability culture we reviewed in Chapter 2, also proposed a popular model of disability identity development. Disabled people tend to be the only members of their family with a disability, which means they generally have no ready access to role (i.e., identity) models. Gill (1997) observed that this reality posed a barrier for feeling and establishing connections to the disability community. This model is a straightforward, stage-based one that identifies four types of integration of disability identity through the lifespan (both congenital and acquired disabilities are accounted for by the model's theoretical base). Gill refers to the stages as "types," but they function in a similar manner.

Integration Type One: Coming to Feel We Belong

The first stage is about becoming integrated into society while having a disability. Here, disabled people recognize that they deserve inclusion with the general public, so they refuse to be segregated or excluded from mainstream culture or activities due to their disabilities. This stage is about recognizing the importance of civil rights, including the need to request accommodations and to seek opportunities that afford greater accessibility. Gill (1997) recognized that integration in this stage will vary by age; older disabled people grew up when the United States did not provide many civil rights to the disabled, while younger people do not know a world without the Americans with Disabilities Act (ADA) and related legislation, as well as medical-technological advances designed to help with the demands of daily life.

Integration Type Two: Coming Home

Becoming integrated with the larger disability community is the goal of the second stage. Here, disabled individuals begin to seek out contact with other disabled people, doing so for support, connection, and shared understanding (particularly among those who have the same condition). When disabled peers join one another, disability culture develops through collective integration. In the past, disabled individuals often avoided contacting their peers due to past segregation and isolation (e.g., medical "warehousing"), memories of stigmatization, and generally being rejected by the nondisabled world.

Integration Type Three: Coming Together

This stage entails the internal integration of recognizing the "sameness" of disability as shared with other disabled people while also acknowledging one's own "difference" or unique disability. Coming together allows younger disabled people to develop favorable attitudes toward their disabilities, which promotes self-acceptance.

TABLE 5.2

Other Representative Theories of Identity Development

Theory	Reference(s)
Livneh's model of adaptation to disability	Livneh, 1986
Charmaz's studies of disabled men	Charmaz 1994, 1995
Disability identity and activist's attitudes	Hahn & Beaulaurier, 2001; Hahn & Belt, 2004
Political disability identity	Putnam, 2005
Weeber's positional model	Weeber, 2004
Gibson's disability identity model	Gibson, 2006
Caldwell's disability identity themes	Caldwell, 2011
Orientation toward disability	Darling, 2013
Narrative approach to disability identity	Dunn & Burcaw, 2013

Source: Adapted from Andrews (2020)

A challenge is that outsiders often try to impose particular goals on insiders that are designed to somehow compensate for the nature of the individuals' disabilities. Thus, someone with a physical disability might be encouraged to avoid recreational activities that require bodily exertion in favor of intellectual pursuits (or vice versa). To navigate these social and psychological pressures, disabled people must claim disability as a key part of the self and identity to avoid conflicted feelings, while also denying outsider perspectives that hide, neglect, or even defame disability (Gill, 1997).

Integration Type Four: Coming Out

This fourth and final stage involves integrating how disabled people feel with the ways they present themselves to the world. In the ideal, a person's private and public selves accept and celebrate their own disability while avoiding the need to seek any form of nondisabled "passing" or the misplaced desire for outsider normalcy (Gill, 1997). Coming out is about living an authentic and honest life with a disability, one that promotes an integrated sense of self, not in isolation but in solidarity with the larger disabled community.

A variety of other disability identity models exist. Examples and accompanying references are found in Table 5.2. Detailed discussion of these and other models may be found in Andrews (2020). We now turn to an increasingly important construct linked to adjustment—disability identity.

Understanding Disability Identity

> Disability identity is a frequently used but imprecisely defined concept . . . [but] there is general agreement that people experiencing disability often feel affinity, or even solidarity, with other[s] who also experience disability.
>
> —Michelle Putnam (2005, p. 188)

Presumably, disability identity emerges from identity development. Wright (1983) wrote that "the self-picture is an intricate one, consisting of a variety of particular characteristics that define for the person his or her *identity*, as well as a global self-evaluation of personal worth" (p. 210, italics in original). The term "disability identity" refers to positive and beneficial perspectives concerning one's own disability while at the same time having close ties to other members of the disability community (e.g., Dunn, 2015; Dunn & Burcaw, 2013; Forber-Pratt et al., in press; Gill, 1997; Olkin & Pledger, 2003). As already implied, disability identity runs on a continuum where people at one pole define themselves by their disabilities while those at the other end downplay, ignore, or even hide their disability status from others and themselves. As already noted, a variety of other possible degrees of disability identity—including some marked by mixed or ambivalent feelings—fall along the continuum.

Identities do enable people to make sense of how they think and feel about themselves (Oyserman et al., 2012). We might expect that while disability identity is defined as containing a positive framework for understanding and even sharing the experience of disability, it is likely that negative information—awareness of stigma, prejudice, stereotypes, and even discrimination or being treated as "the other"—is there, as well. Thus, disability identity allows for recognition of social control as espoused by outsiders but also the opportunity to advance social change by and for insiders (Siebers, 2011). A working disability identity can help to guide a disabled individual to know how to respond in situations where a disability might suddenly become salient. More to the point, the members of any minority group, including one as large and as heterogeneous as the disability community, do not have to personally experience prejudice to recognize it (Dunn, 2015).

Depending on the circumstance, the presence of a disability identity could elicit positive or negative reactions, so that the individual's subsequent behavior could be self-affirming or problematic. Social psychological research on stereotype threat, for example, could be relevant here. *Stereotype threat* is a psychosocial form of vulnerability, one where members of groups experience behavioral challenges (e.g., academic skills, athletic ability, social poise) when their performance is tied to biased opinions or prevailing (if usually erroneous) expectations (Steele, 1997, 2011). White males, for example, can underperform when reminded of the stereotype that people of Asian descent are believed to be more highly skilled at quantitative problem solving (Aronson et al., 1999). Due to self-imposed cognitive pressure or distraction, they may receive lower test scores when they are reminded of the stereotype (e.g., "This math test measures innate quantitative reasoning skills.") than when the directive is more neutral (e.g., "This is a measure of general knowledge."), so that the predominant group stereotype is not activated in their memories.

In the case of disability, we would assume that disabled individuals could become self-conscious in some circumstances (e.g., trying to get to a social event in a building that does not appear to have conveniently located elevators), so that they assume that their search triggers stereotyped responses from observers (e.g., "Wheelchair users cannot fend for themselves"). In such cases, the weight of stereotype threat could lead to behaviors indicative of poor coping, such as expressed frustration or dependence on others. If nothing else, insiders could be distracted by their imaginings of what watchful outsiders are thinking. Yet disability identity is only *one* aspect of an individual's identity—depending on the situation, another identity, or other identities (e.g., spouse, parent, employer, friend, neighbor, mentor), might supersede its influence.

We do know that people tell stories about their experiences, including those that are disability-related. Sometimes, such stories are narrative representations of how people with congenital or acquired disabilities have adjusted to them. In a recent memoir, *Easy Beauty*, the philosopher Chloe' Cooper Jones (2022) wrote about the fact that her new acquaintances are often moved to ask about the origin of her disability (which is sacral agenesis); they tend to assume she acquired some disease or befell some accident instead of being born with her condition, as she was. They prefer a "normal" before and a "not good" after. One problem is that all her life these before and after expectations offered by others shaped her sense of self. She accepted these expectations because she found some people were more likely to accept her as she is if she did.

Hevern (2008, p. 218) suggested that stories like those found in *Easy Beauty* advance goals the authors value, including

- Attaching meaning to their ongoing experiences
- Predicting how key actors (themselves, others) will behave in the future
- Allowing negotiation with or navigation through various social worlds
- Establishing personal identities for themselves and for other people

TABLE 5.3

Key Themes Representative of Disability Identity Drawn from Narratives

Communal attachment: Desire and feeling to affiliate with other persons with disabilities
Affirmation of disability: Private thoughts and feelings of inclusion in the larger social order, possessing the same rights and responsibilities as other citizens
Self-worth: Valuing the self with a disability; feeling equal to nondisabled people
Pride: Being proud of one's identity while also recognizing that disability is a quality devalued by the nondisabled majority
Discrimination: Awareness of self and other disabled persons as targets of prejudiced thoughts, feelings, and behaviors in daily life
Personal meaning: Finding significance, making sense, and identifying benefits associated with disability

Source: Adapted from Dunn and Burcaw (2013)

This last goal is relevant for the present discussion, though the others matter, too. Dunn and Burcaw (2013) reviewed some published narratives authored by disabled persons about their experiences and lives. To do so, the investigators relied on a thematic model of inquiry (e.g., Riessman, 2008) to categorize their narrative samples using themes identified as representative of disability identity. Table 5.3 presents six key themes discerned from their narrative samples. Two themes—*communal attachment* and *affirmation of disability*—deal with qualities of disability identity that represent civil protest and activism as well as ties to disability culture (e.g., Gill, 1997; Hahn & Belt, 2004). The subsequent three themes—*self-worth*, *pride*, and *discrimination* are found in research on disability politics and activism (e.g., Putnam, 2005). The final theme—*personal meaning*—is related to the personal acceptance of one's disability (Dunn & Burcaw, 2013; Wright, 1983). Narratives written by disabled authors were the source of the themes (for a list of the memoirs used in the study, please see Dunn & Burcaw, 2013). There is little doubt that a different set of narratives might reveal additional key themes, and in fact, narratives usually contain more than one disability identity theme.

Dunn and Burcaw (2013) suggest that practitioners could share relevant narratives with recently disabled clients to draw parallels to their own experience. Similarly, narratives can be used to demonstrate positive coping following the onset of disability. Caregivers, family members, and friends might also benefit from reading some narratives so that they can become sensitive to the issues potentially affecting their disabled person. Finally, with careful guidance, some disabled individuals might be encouraged to write their own disability identity stories to reflect on disability more deeply and personally. Social psychological research finds that such self-narratives serve constructive purposes as people seek to develop positive outlooks and behaviors (e.g., Walton & Wilson, 2018; Wilson, 2011) or navigate negative life events (e.g., Pennebaker, 1997, 2004).

What about whether a disability is congenital or acquired? Does either status influence one's disability identity? Bogart (2014) demonstrated differences among adults with congenital rather than acquired disabilities—namely, that the former displayed higher disability identification and life satisfaction scores than the latter. Relying on a modified version of the Acceptance of Disability Scale (Linkowski, 1971), a sample of people with congenital disabilities reported greater acceptance of disability than did a group with acquired conditions (Li & Moore, 1998). Using an international sample, Nario-Redmond and Oleson (2016) showed that disability identity was highest among individuals who had been living with disability for a greater proportion of their lives. Another US sample found that people with more visible conditions scored higher on disability identification than those whose disabilities remained "hidden unless disclosed" (Nario-Redmond et al., 2013). Darling and Heckert (2010) showed that the presence of a congenital disability was a strong predictor of positive disability identity; such participants described higher levels of disability pride, while those who acquired their disabilities later in life associated greater shame with their conditions. The passage of time since the onset of disability was also positively correlated with pride in being disabled (Darling & Heckert, 2010).

Recently, disability affirmation and acceptance were found to be predictive of hope among adults with physical disabilities; however, the presence of multiple disabilities was negatively related to the individuals' agency (Zapata, 2020). Previously, Bat-Chava (1994) tracked a strong sense of group connection and identity among the Deaf to higher levels of self-esteem, but this finding does not always emerge among specific impairment groups, including those with cognitive or learning disabilities (Finlay & Lyons, 1998).

Although disability identity is a promising area for investigation, there is much we do not know about the construct. Where the influence of congenital versus acquired disabilities is concerned, for example, the available cross-sectional studies are suggestive, but their conclusions are not definitive. As Forber-Pratt et al. (2017) observed, most published work relies on small sample sizes (many with fewer than 10 participants), and only a couple of studies have more than 100 participants (see DePape & Lindsay, 2015; Raskind et al., 2006). Many of these studies are based on rich, qualitative self-reports, but their generalizability is suspect. There are no studies that fully explore the purported favorable qualities that comprise disability identify, notably the presumed connection to the disability community. Perhaps future investigators will be spurred to undertake the necessary longitudinal research to fully explore this compelling construct. For more discussions of disability identity, see Andrews (2020), Bogart and Nario-Redman (2019), Dunn (2015), and Forber-Pratt et al. (in press). As Olkin and Pledger (2003, p. 302) observed some time ago,

> Although it might be hypothesized that disability identity and feeling a part of the disability community are buffers against the stresses of being an oppressed minority, this has not been directly examined.... Is identity a buffer against... disability-specific hassles?

Other Evidence for Positive Adjustment to Disability

Besides disability formation and identity, there are other examples that point to favorable adjustment to disability. We will briefly consider two of them: resilience and finding positive meaning following a disability. Other examples can be found in Wehmeyer and Dunn (2022) and Andrews et al. (in press).

RESILIENCE

Perhaps due to continued interest in positive psychology, resilience has become a popular psychological topic. *Resilience* is defined as an ability to adapt to and return from adverse circumstances (Dunn, 2022; Dunn & Ayers, in press). In the popular mind, resilience is presumed to be relatively rare and a matter of one's personality or innate drive; in reality, neither of these views is valid (Bonanno, 2012). Resilience is generally considered a dynamic and multidimensional process, which can spawn a variety of different approaches to respond and adjust to misfortune. Most individuals who encounter adversity (e.g., awful accidents, private traumas, natural disasters, disabling experiences)—around two-thirds of them—rise above the situation and flourish, while the remainder founder and often suffer (e.g., Bonanno & Diminich, 2013; Galatzer-Levy et al., 2018). Resilient people respond in particularly adaptive ways; key qualities are how they appraise, understand, and then cope with the encountered stressors. Unlike nonresilient others, they are more accepting of what is happening to them and generally perceive less threat to their well-being (Masten et al., 2009). Their coping efforts, too, are more active and engaged, displaying higher levels of efficacy than those who show other adjustment patterns (e.g., Quale & Schanke, 2010).

At present, not much research has focused on resilience and its relationship to disability (Terrill et al., 2019). According to the WHO International Classification of Functioning, Disability, and Heath (ICF) model, resilience can be an *intrapersonal factor* or a quality that either resides in or is developed following the onset of disability (see Chapter 1). Terrill and colleagues highlighted coping styles, positive emotions, meaning making (which will be discussed shortly), and optimism. Social psychological research on disability, in turn, indicates that resilience can emerge from *situational factors*—say, when some variable outside the person interacts with or possibly triggers some personal qualities (e.g., Dunn, 2015; Wright, 1983). One such situation-specific construct that can promote resilience is self-efficacy, or knowing what or how to do something and being confident that it can be done (Terrill et al., 2019).

How can resilience be promoted among the recently disabled? One study examined how adhering to one's values following spinal cord injury (SCI) was found to be associated with higher levels of resilience. In a study conducted by Kuzu et al. (2024), values reflecting altruism and prosocial attitudes were found among sample members who showed high resilience. Perhaps identifying personal values and setting goals for a more value-based life—where one would be focused on caring for and helping other people—can heighten resilience among those who experience a SCI. The key may be to identify those who can intentionally live by their values, as high-resilience participants rated values including compassion, caring, gratitude, contribution, respect, and responsibility as significantly more important than those showing low resilience. Of course, these results are suggestive but preliminary, and more research on the role of values is needed.

At this juncture, resilience is presumed to be a central construct linked to adjusting to disability, though consistently convincing data are lacking. Interested disability researchers should address the problem of most studies being cross-sectional and thereby failing to track the multisystemic processes of resilience present in daily life and across time (Mesman et al., 2021). As Dunn and Ayers (in press) observed, the de facto measurement of resilience is based on self-report measures emphasizing coping and self-regulation. Assessment also needs to determine the effect of the potential instability of various physical and social ecological systems on resilience, including the impact of ableism and other forms of sociopolitical oppression. An improved and broader understanding of resilience will enhance the effectiveness of interventions designed to promote positive outcomes for disabled individuals.

We now consider another form of positive outcome: finding positive meaning in disabling experiences.

FINDING POSITIVE MEANING IN DISABILITY

Various investigators argue that one consequence of experiencing a loss, trauma, or disabling event is the search for meaning (e.g., Frankl, 1985; Janoff-Bulman, 1992). More to the point, better and more complete adaptation to changed circumstances is possible when people discern positive meaning in their adversity (e.g., Keany & Glueckauf, 1993; Schulz & Decker, 1985; Taylor et al., 1984; Thompson & Janigian, 1988; Vash & Crewe, 2004). The search for benefits or "silver linings" in otherwise negative circumstances enables the affected individuals to impose a framework of coherence on what happened to them (e.g., Antonovsky, 1987). Some researchers also suggest that discerning positive meaning in an otherwise bleak situation enables people to do better physically and emotionally, so that successful adjustment can be posited (e.g., Collins et al., 1990; Tait & Silver, 1989).

One important aspect of disability onset is that those affected ask and try to answer questions regarding why this circumstance befell them and not someone else. This matters because it involves attending to—and granting credence to—subjective human experiences (Wegner & Gilbert, 2000) and how people construe events in their lives (Wilson, 2022). Thus, self-reports of positive adjustment and coping still need to be evaluated critically and with empirical validation whenever feasible, but they should not be discounted as "wishful thinking" or some form of dissonance reduction.

Dunn (1996) explored well-being following amputation in a group of 138 amputee golfers (the average time since limb loss in the sample was just over 20 years), and most of the amputations were due to trauma or disease and trauma combined; a few were due to congenital conditions. Using a mailed survey, the golfers completed standard depression and self-esteem measures and a measure of dispositional optimism and then were asked whether they found any positive meaning linked to and perceived control over their disability. Those who found positive meaning after their amputations had lower levels of depressive symptoms than those who did not. Those with higher levels of optimism and greater perceived control over their disability also had lower depression scores and reported higher levels of self-esteem. The participants' reported examples of positive meaning were categorized according to attribution types found in the relevant social psychological literature (see Table 5.4). In a sense, if a person finds some positive meaning, the category or attribution type does not matter—favorable adjustment is linked to the found meaning.

Meaningfulness clearly matters to humans, and it may help them to adjust to radical life changes and challenges (Baumeister & Vohs, 2002). As Elliott et al. (2002) noted,

TABLE 5.4

Positive Meaning Examples Following Amputation by Attribution Type

Reframed event positively
"All good has come out of it."
"I found God through it."
"It has given me purpose."
"It makes me special."
Engaged in social comparison
"I have one leg. What about the person who has no legs?"
Imagined worse situations
"I survived. I have a second chance at life. I love it."
Found side benefits
"I changed to a different occupation [where] I became very successful."
Forgot negative aspects
"I found that I can still do about everything I did before—only it takes me longer to do it."

Source: Adapted from Dunn (1996, p. 291, Table 1)

> Most observers have overlooked the potentially valuable experience of acquiring a physical disability. Writers have given only scant attention to positive growth and optimal living with chronic health problems, as well as the related searches for meaning, purpose, and fulfillment (p. 687).

Precis and Prospects

The third foundational principle, *adjustment to disability*, is assumed to be a dynamic process that varies from person to person. Adjustment can follow adaptation and sometimes acceptance of a disability. Yet there is no one way to adjust to a disabling life event, and some individuals never do. Indeed, disability is one adverse event that may permanently alter people's set point of subjective well-being, though this does not mean that people who acquire a disability lead troubled lives. Adjustment can emerge from identity formation processes and a positive disability identity. There is some evidence that those with congenital disabilities show better adjustment than those who acquire them later in life, but more evidence is needed. Resilience and finding positive meaning are two other modes that can promote favorable adjustment to disability. In Chapter 6, we will learn about the importance of psychological assets, the personal or psychological qualities a person already has or can acquire to undo challenges posed by disability while also enhancing daily life.

THOUGHT QUESTIONS

1. What is *adjustment* to disability? How does it relate to or differ from *adaptation* and *acceptance*?
2. Do all people with disabilities (whether congenital or acquired) eventually adjust to their conditions? Why or why not?
3. What is the *hedonic treadmill* metaphor, and how does it apply to how people adjust to good or bad events? Does the hedonic treadmill apply to the experience of disability?
4. Has interest in positive psychology influenced the study of adjustment to disability? How so?
5. What are the stages of Gill's model of disability identity formation? Does this model characterize the experience of all disabled persons? Why or why not?
6. Define disability identity. How is disability identity hypothesized to influence adjustment to disability or other chronic health conditions?
7. Can narrative approaches to the examination of disability identity aid those with congenital or acquired disabilities?
8. Resilience is believed to be another psychosocial construct that promotes adjustment: What is it, and how is it believed to help disabled people cope with the onset of disability?
9. Why do many people seem to find positive meaning after a disabling event? How can finding meaning promote psychosocial adjustment to disability?

6 Principle 4

PSYCHOLOGICAL ASSETS

Foundational Principle 4: Psychological assets

People with disabilities possess or can acquire personal or psychological qualities that can ameliorate challenges posed by disability and also enrich daily living

> One can appreciate the asset value of something without purposely invoking a comparative standard, as when one enjoys a balmy evening or a musical performance because of the pleasure one gets from their inherent qualities, not because they are better or worse than something to which they are compared. In the same way, one can value the functional usefulness of a prothesis or wheelchair without putting them down as less functional than the intact body.
>
> —Beatrice A. Wright (1983, p. 180)

> This Foundational Principle highlights the potential array of resources that are distinctive in each person and can be a point of pride during or after a rehabilitation experience.
>
> —Dunn et al. (2016, p. 3)

In a discussion of how disabled people's values can change, Wright (1983) described how the known attributes of a person (e.g., appearance, attractiveness, abilities, background) could represent "status implications" for an observer evaluating them.

On the Foundational Principles of Rehabilitation Psychology. Dana S. Dunn, Oxford University Press.
 DOI: 10.1093/9780197785188.003.0006

As Wright put it, "The attributes in question may be said to have status value for the evaluator, and the evaluator may be said to invoke status values" (p. 179). Such *status values* trigger comparisons with some standard ranging from (in theory) better to worse or positive to negative, and they have also been labeled *comparative values* (see Dembo et al., 1956). Wright noted that in the case of other different evaluators, the same values might not be viewed as having any status dimensions at all. When this happens, the values are evaluated using other metrics, such as their utility for the person or their intrinsic worth. Then the focus is on the nature or function of the attribute and not on the individual's position relative to that of other people. This form of evaluation enables a given attribute to be perceived as an asset that, where status judgments are concerned, would be coded as below standard. Here, however, it is referred to as an *asset evaluation*, and the values tied to it become *asset values*. Why does this analysis matter in the context of disability? A person's ability to use a cane, walker, prosthetic limb, or wheelchair can be seen as an asset, one that need not be devalued, seen as devaluing, or in any way representing their status as an inferior one.

Yet when status judgments occur, the standard for comparison is usually an imagined average; to be regarded as worthy of induction into an honor society, for example, one ought to have certain accomplishments to be invited to join the ranks. In this and other real or imagined situations, whether the person is deemed worthy is a judgment of their status. American culture is rife with social comparison (Festinger, 1954), much of which is about status comparisons (e.g., occupation, education, car, clothing, salary, title). Yet Wright (1983) believed that asset evaluations happen regularly, though they may not be recognized: "Friends often relate to each other without the distorting lens of status comparisons (p. 179)." When competition in such relations appears, the friendship may struggle or even falter.

Where disability is concerned, Wright (1983) wanted to reduce or even eliminate using status comparisons due to their damaging nature and their focus on comparative loss or "what used to be." In contrast, asset values can be perceived as very important but will not necessarily elicit self-judgments of relative standing or personal worth. High asset value can be placed on certain activities, such as watching a play, listening to music, visiting a park or garden, reading, and so on. All of these are good things to do or enjoy, but they are not necessarily devaluing if they are not currently available to you (i.e., we may not visit a park in foul weather; we can listen to a book instead of reading it).

Following a disabling event, part of the process of adjustment (recall Chapter 5) is focusing on what can be accomplished or done in a different way, that is, recognizing the activity's asset or intrinsic value. The affected person (now an insider) can value what can be done without comparing how it is done by others (i.e., outsiders). Wright argued that disabled individuals can experience psychological gains when asset values are not turned into comparison values. When they are, time and energy are wasted and comparative disappointments (what cannot be done) replace an asset (what can be done) focus (for a related discussion, see Marini & Villarreal, 2024). Certainly, as the process of adjustment to disability advances, favorable adaptation is linked to recognizing already possessed assets or seeking new ones rather than ruing comparisons with the past.[1]

Having established the theory behind asset value, let's explore the sorts of assets people with disabilities possess.

Identifying and Understanding Assets

One of the implications of the fourth foundational principle is this: No matter how severe a disability might turn out to be, every disabled individual is assumed to either possess or have the capacity to develop some asset or assets. Assets are part and parcel of the wide variety of resources that are hypothesized to exist in all people, including one's self-identity or self-concept; particular strengths or personal qualities; physical, social, intellectual, or professional capacities; and career or work-related aptitudes. Many assets are apparent, like the social support one receives from family and friends or the security provided by one's income or residence. Others are earned or attainable (e.g., job or profession, awards and honors, education), imagined (e.g., dreams, hopes) or enacted (e.g., goals), or even personality-based (e.g., optimism, extraversion, wit) or motivationally driven (e.g., persistence, self-discipline). An asset can be an esoteric interest (e.g., the history of ancient Rome, the philosophy of Hegel, the songs of Sinatra), a hobby (e.g., photography, collecting antiques, gardening), or prosocial activities (e.g., volunteer work, community service). "Remaining resources" is the term applied to any assets that people retain following the onset of disability or chronic illness (Vash & Crewe, 2004), which will naturally vary from person to person. Some asset categories—with supporting examples underneath each—are shown in Table 6.1. The entries in Table 6.1 are by no means exhaustive, as readers can readily imagine others that could be listed.

As shown by Table 6.1, assets can be real, perceived, potential, personal, hidden, or acquired. Their presence is the means for an individual to present, develop, and maintain a clear identity, as well as to display familiar social roles (e.g., parent,

1. In the case of congenital disabilities, there is no real adjustment period or process, so individuals learn what they need to do by adapting to or changing aspects of their environments (recall foundational principle 1; see Chapter 3).

TABLE 6.1

Asset Categories with Supporting Examples
Family
Spouse or partner
Parent or child
Sibling or relative
Education
High school graduate or GED
Associate or bachelor's degree
Graduate degree
Social Support
Family
Friends
Coworkers or colleagues
Neighborhood
Religious community
Job/work/career
Full- or part-time employment
Income
Expertise, training, or specialization
Finances/income
Stable income
Retirement account or pension
Home ownership
Personality and learnable qualities
Optimism
Extraversion
Abilities (e.g., delay gratification, express gratitude)
Character strengths and virtues
Goal setting
Recreation
Hobbies and pastimes
Sports (as participant or fan)
Travel

TABLE 6.1 *Continued*

Spirituality
Faith
Membership in church, temple, synagogue, mosque
Community
Volunteer
Community service
Mentor to youth
Board member

Source: Adapted from in Dunn (2015, Table 2.2)

child, spouse). Assets also allow people to express their vocations or avocations, both to themselves and to others. An asset can illustrate a solitary interest or pursuit (e.g., drawing, painting) or a collective one with social elements (e.g., golf, board games). When assets are present and apparent, they communicate the fact that a disabled person is doing *something*. They can also be opportunities, as is the case when disabled individuals decide to learn a new activity, take up a new hobby, or receive new training. Thus, assets can be motivational, promoting those with disabilities to be action-oriented and perhaps even resilient (Craig, 2012; Dunn, 2022; Dunn, Uswatte, & Elliott, 2021) in their given situations. Naturally, encouragement to maintain existing assets or to acquire new ones should emanate from family, caregivers, friends, and medical and rehabilitation professionals (e.g., Tackett et al., 2016), as well as the insiders themselves (e.g., Nierenberg et al., 2016).

The examination of assets also aligns with an important set of constructs from positive psychology. Peterson and Seligman (2004) created a detailed organization of what they called character strengths and virtues. These favorable, individual traits were organized into the Values in Action (VIA) Classification of Strengths, a positive alternative to the well-known but pathology-focused *Diagnostic and Statistical Manual of Mental Disorders* (DSM). The Values in Action Inventory of Strengths (VIA-IS) measures 24 strengths that fall into six domains: wisdom and knowledge (e.g., love of learning), courage (e.g., integrity), humanity (e.g., love), justice (e.g., fairness), temperance (e.g., modesty), and transcendence (e.g., hope). Individuals can use this instrument to identify their current strengths and to possibly leverage them in ways that enhance their everyday lives while also promoting their personal well-being (Peterson & Park, 2011). What makes these character strengths and virtues different than, say, personality traits, is that they represent assets that can be learned (Niemiec, 2013; Peterson & Seligman, 2004), including following a disabling event. In addition, they can also contribute to a sense of meaningfulness in life (recall Chapter 5; see Peterson & Park 2012).

We need to recognize that the onset of disability or chronic illness can contribute to the reduction in capacity or even loss of an asset. As noted at the outset of this chapter, the risk is that an individual will compare their prior state of being with their postdisability state of being—potentially into a status or comparative value, with accompanying negativity. While quite human, emphasizing the loss of an asset (e.g., "I'll never be able to do *x* again") should be avoided, as it is demoralizing, counterproductive, and not always accurate. As already acknowledged, disability is a process and not an end state; adjustment, too, is dynamic, different for everyone, and something that happens across time. It is possible that an asset can be relearned or done in a different way—or that a new asset can replace the previous one. Some therapeutic value lies in helping recently disabled persons to reframe their experience by comparing their current self with their soon-after-disability-onset self; distance from the event (becoming disabled) may lead to new perspectives and adjustment (being disabled). In any case, whether a disability is newly acquired, established, or congenital, the focus should always be on what can be achieved, learned, relearned, or done in a new way. As Wright (1983) advocated, disabled persons may need to adjust their values or adopt new ones and thereby revise their assets, goals, and priorities to fit their evolving experiences rather than dwelling on what once was. Doing so is not always an easy feat, but one way to try is to help clients determine for themselves what qualities make a life with or after disability.

The Good Life and Disability: Definition and an Asset Focus

What is or makes for a good life? What is a good life with disability like? How do assets affect the nature of a good life living with a disability or other chronic illness?

To begin, we must be aware that living with a disability potentially leads to unique pleasures as well as challenges that are distinct from living a life without such a constraint (e.g., McBryde Johnson, 2005). At the same time, we want to also steer clear of inadvertently making value judgments—especially those based on status or comparative values that might suggest what disabled individuals *must do* (or *avoid* doing) to improve their lives and sense of well-being (for consideration of the perceived risks of such value judgments in general, see Csikszentmihalyi, 2006). Autonomy, choice, and self-direction matter. We need to remember that a disability only affects selective slices of daily life—not the whole—so it should be regarded as one influence among many in people's ongoing experiences. Still, what do we mean by *a* or *the* good life?

WHAT IS THE GOOD LIFE?

Describing, defining, or delineating the nature or composition of "the good life" is one of the preoccupations of philosophers, theologians, and poets and, of late, psychologists (e.g., Bauer, 2021; Baumeister et al., 2013; Csikszentmihalyi, 2021; Dunn & Brody, 2008; Kukita et al., 2022; O'Brien et al., 2018). Can thoughts, choices, and behaviors lead us there? Laypersons, too, want to know "how to live" to be happy or at least content. Given the stresses and strains of contemporary life, finding an answer or a behavioral solution to the problem makes sense. Lots of possibilities have been floated, including work, wealth, friendship, love, health, education, security, and leisure time, to account for what might constitute the good life (e.g., Wilson, 2008). In the positive psychology literature, money was discounted as a likely source because it did not seem to enhance happiness once a certain salary level was met (around $75,000.00 per year; see Kahneman & Deaton, 2010), but the finding was later proven to be in error—incrementally speaking, earning more money does lead to higher contentment and well-being (Killingsworth, 2021; Killingsworth et al., 2023).[2]

In ancient Greek philosophy, for example, three variants of the good life one might seek were identified (Craig, 1998a). Ordered from most to least favorable, they include an introspective, self-aware, and philosophically based existence; a politically focused but virtuous life (i.e., helping the state and its citizens); and a hedonistic life tied to profit making and material acquisition. Presumably, individuals followed the third variant only if they did not recognize the personal fulfillment to be found in a contemplative or service-oriented life. The Greeks, then, believed that the good life was grounded in the pursuit of *eudaimonia*, a term that roughly means "flourishing" or "happiness." However, this traditional notion of happiness is distinct from our more self-oriented variation (e.g., Ryan & Deci, 2001; Waterman, 1993). Our sense of happiness tends to be short in duration and linked to a past, current, or anticipated (future) event (e.g., "My college graduation day was a happy one." "This is a great concert." "I can't wait for my vacation."). Our happiness is also a subjective state of being, one where an individual's overall experience is satisfactory ("All things considered, I'm generally pretty happy.").

2. The exception occurs when people are rich but miserable, so that more money will not elevate their happiness—and a subset of very wealthy people are like that (see Berger, 2023).

In contrast, *eudaimonia* was construed to be a more objective state, one representing the greatest possible good—a life of contentment based on doing well by living well and pursuing a contemplative life (Craig, 1998b). Ethics, too, mattered. To lead a good life, developing and exercising virtues was important, so that autonomy, individual growth, and self-acceptance were clearly present (Ryff, 1989; Ryff & Singer, 2008). There was little room for pursuing material wealth or bodily pleasures—reason and reflection were the point. Pleasure for its own sake was frowned upon.

How did conceptions of the good life evolve across time? During the medieval period, philosophers believed that the good life represented seeking the "highest good" or, in Latin, the *summum bonum*; that is, becoming and remaining a virtuous person by pursing—and displaying—virtues. It was assumed that virtuous individuals could intuitively recognize the "good" (Audi, 1995). By the 20th century, Moore (1971), a prominent moral philosopher, argued that the good life is recognized when innately satisfying states and actions occur, such as appreciating beauty, becoming learned or knowledgeable, and taking pleasure in friendship. The tenets of this moral philosophy are more or less commensurate with current psychology's understanding of the good life.

POSITIVE PSYCHOLOGY'S TAKE ON THE GOOD LIFE

Since its beginning in the late 1990s, positive psychologists have been interested in understanding and building on the things that people do well, which means trying to define the good life in contemporary terms (perhaps with the occasional nod to historical precedents). Three elements were identified as promoting the good life: positive connections to others, positive personal qualities, and life regulation qualities (e.g., Bolt & Dunn, 2016; Compton, 2004; Dunn & Brody, 2008; Seligman, 2002; Snyder & Lopez, 2002; Snyder et al., 2021). We will briefly review each element in turn and see that assets can be a part of each element precisely because they are flexible and mutable.

Positive Connections to Others

As social beings, humans generally seek to form favorable relationships with other people. Such connections exist when people possess the requisite social skills to form and maintain friendships, as well as when they express love for others (whether family or friends) or forgive people's wrongdoings or other lapses in judgment. These and related sorts of assets could be found under "Family," "Social Support," and "Community" in Table 6.1.

Positive Personal Qualities

These are represented by individuals' abilities to express gratitude, to be creative, and to demonstrate discipline, among other character traits. Some of these traits originate in people's personalities, while others can be learned. Assets tied to such positive qualities could appear under "Personality and Learnable Qualities" in Table 6.1.

Life Regulation Qualities

Such qualities allow people to be autonomous and self-controlled while pursuing goals that influence the lives of those who are close to them or dependent upon them. Are they able to delay immediate gratification to plan for their futures? Can they commit the time to learn new skills necessary to complete important tasks? Personality and learnable qualities contain these and related sorts of assets; depending on the situation, related assets also might be found under "Family," "Social Support," "Job/Work/Career," and "Spirituality, and Community" (see Table 6.1). The social venues found within these categories all shape people's behavior, attitudes, and outlooks. And, of course, other influential categories exist that do not appear in Table 6.1 because they are more idiosyncratic and tied to individuals' unique life experiences (this is also true for other *positive connections to others* and *positive personal qualities*). Rehabilitation psychologists, medical professionals, and counseling therapists need to keep this fact in mind when helping clients identify, articulate, and focus on their assets or would-be assets. (We will return to reflect on more asset examples in each of the three identified categories at the end of this chapter.)

Based on a review of the literature pertaining to predicting happiness, subjective well-being, life satisfaction, and related positive constructs, Dunn and Brody (2008) identified variables that do and do not predict consistent associations with the good life (whether one is disabled or not). As we will see, few of these factors have pronounced effects on people's well-being at the aggregate level. We will briefly discuss these factors and then consider them in light of their potential therapeutic importance as assets following the onset of disability or some other chronic illness. For a more detailed discussion of these predictor variables and their influence on positive or negative states, please see, for example, Diener and Diener (1996), Diener et al. (1999), Dunn and Brody (2008), Eid and Larsen (2008), and Kahneman et al. (1999).

Table 6.2 list some variables that often have a strong connection to the positive states that are defined as comprising the good life (Dunn & Brody, 2008). Note that the top of the table shows positive predictors linked to individual circumstance as well as individual differences. Regarding the former, being employed,

TABLE 6.2

Positive and Negative Variables with Stronger Predictive Associations with the Good Life

Individual circumstance	Individual differences
Positive predictors	
Employment	Frequency of experiencing positive affect
Frequency of sexual intercourse	Ability to express gratitude
Frequency of experiencing positive affect	Being optimistic
Income[a]	Higher self-esteem
Negative predictors	
Divorced	
Widow or widower	
Unemployment	
Disability	

[a] Income is included in this table due to the research done by Killingsworth (2021) and Killingsworth et al. (2023), which was discussed earlier in this chapter.
Source: Adapted from Dunn & Brody (2008, Table 2, p. 416)

having the opportunity for sex, experiencing positive emotions regularly (due to eliciting situations), and having a higher income are associated with the good life. The latter, personality-related factors, again involve the frequency of experiencing positive affect (some people are constitutionally more prone to do so than others), being grateful, being optimistic, and having higher levels of self-esteem. The bottom section of Table 6.2 lists circumstantial predictor variables that are often associated with negative states (i.e., lower reported well-being, happiness, or life satisfaction). Divorce reduces happiness, as does the death of a spouse and being unemployed; however, though it can last for a long period of time, such reduced happiness or well-being is rarely permanent. Disability is also one of these variables and, as acknowledged earlier, it can sometimes reduce positive states perpetually. Although not all forms of disability are likely linked to negative states (e.g., as you will recall, congenital disabilities are often an exception), some are, as was discussed in Chapter 5 with respect to psychosocial adjustment, as well as the so-called hedonic treadmill.

As shown in Table 6.3, a wide variety of variables have no or a very low correlational association with the good life (see the first column in the table). Intuitively and certainly anecdotally, many of these factors would seem to logically predict a good life—like the more education one has or if one is physically attractive, has children, or lives in a temperate or ideal part of the United States (i.e., climate zone). While

TABLE 6.3

Other Variables and Their Level of Predictive Association with the Good Life

No or Low Correlation	Individual Differences	Moderate Correlation[a]
Education	Extraversion	Number of close friends
Social Class	Conscientiousness	Religiosity
Intelligence	Internal locus of control	Recreational activities, interests
	(Low) neuroticism	
Age		Physical health
Gender		
Physical attractiveness		
Race/ethnicity		
Having children		
Climate zone		

[a] Being married was originally included in this table as being moderately associated with the good life; however, DePaulo (2015, 2018) argues that the correlation is a potentially spurious one and that the differences between married and single people are small and often need to be qualified. And in any case, we cannot do the experimental research needed to demonstrate cause and effect; that is, we cannot randomly assign some people to marry and some to remain single and so on. Note that the argument is not that marriage is not beneficial (or as we will see, an asset) but, rather, that it may not represent a more favorable state than being single.

Source: Adapted from Dunn & Brody (2008, Table 1, p. 415)

these factors may provide a variety of satisfactions and can readily be perceived to be assets, in and of themselves they do not appear to increase one's incremental happiness in a noticeable manner (though we should also keep in mind that most people are happy—and some are very happy; see Diener & Diener, 1996; Diener & Seligman, 2002). The second column in Table 6.3 lists personality-related factors that are sometimes modestly associated with the good life; therefore, it can be beneficial to be extraverted, to be conscientious, and to believe you can make things happen (high level of internal locus of control), as well as not being anxious (low in neuroticism). Finally, the good life is moderately predictable from having several close friends, being engaged in a religious community, doing recreational activities, and being physically healthy.

Thus, quite a few correlates that would make sense as being predictive of the good life fail to do so. Does this mean such factors do not influence a given person's sense of well-being? No—as Dunn and Brody (2008) observed, "Most people live a moderately good life regardless of how they fare on any of these variables" (p. 415). Rather, we must remember that most of these variables, especially when they are viewed as assets, must be considered contextually. Having children, for example, has no or a low predictive association with happiness, but many, if not most, people would say their children are more than assets in their lives; they are apt to be an essential part of their lives (indeed, see Nelson et al., 2013). Other factors have a more moderate association; for example, the number of close friends one has is predictive of subjective well-being (SWB), and friends are also intuitively as well as obviously an asset. Reliable statistical evidence is important when trying to understand the experiences of many people; however, a more nuanced approach is needed when trying to understand and perhaps improve the outlook of one person who is newly or recently disabled. Professionals, especially therapists, need to point out the benefits tied to existing assets or guide their clients to consider developing new ones.

WHITHER THE GOOD LIFE?

The good life is based not on one thing but on many things, including the assets people already possess or can acquire. Starting in 2010, the late positive psychologist Christopher Peterson maintained a blog on positive psychology for *Psychology Today*'s website. His first 100 online columns (he revised and updated them) were published in a book titled *Pursuing the Good Life* (Peterson, 2013). Although the book was not meant to be a "how to live" book, many, even most, of the short entries can be read that way, and not surprisingly, many of them contain elements that could qualify as assets. For those who want to explore psychosocial assets in a broader way, it may prove to be a good starting point.

We now consider how best to leverage assets in ways that may promote the successful pursuit of happiness.

Unlocking Assets: Intentional Behaviors as Key

One of the challenges posed by our review of approaches to understanding and seeking the good life is using assets in ways that sustain happiness. Research regarding psychosocial adjustment to our circumstances indicates that the hedonic treadmill model often characterizes our affective experiences; although we may experience heightened happiness or well-being, it rarely lasts, and we eventually return to our customary range of feelings. Lyubomirsky et al. (2005) advanced a heuristic model (really, a happiness pie chart) for understanding three major influences on chronic well-being: people's set point of happiness. About 50% is due to genetic factors, 10% is linked to circumstantial factors (which are not very mutable, such as one's family and home environment), and 40% is tied to individuals' volitional or intentional activity factors (or what people choose to do make themselves happier). Lyubomirsky and colleagues argued that the first two components were relatively fixed factors, while the third one allowed people to potentially change how they feel by enacting particular behaviors. For our purposes, assets are implicated in many such behaviors.

Following the appearance of the sustainable happiness model, various researchers identified possible flaws in it (e.g., Bergink, 2015; Brown & Rohrer, 2019; Kashdan, 2015; Krueger, 2015). For example, the percentages attributed to each of the three factors were deemed questionable and perhaps overestimated (see Brown & Rohrer, 2019, for a detailed analysis). Lyubomirsky et al. (2005) never claimed that these estimates were much more than suggested approximations—these authors were mostly focused on advancing the theoretical view that people could affect their own happiness by engaging in intentional behaviors designed to do just that. Sheldon and Lyubomirsky (2021) responded to these critical views by accepting them as useful foils for correcting their speculations and focusing their efforts on developing additional models that could more successfully demonstrate their claims. As we learned earlier, various demographic variables (e.g., gender, race, ethnicity) showed rather small or even nonexistent associations with the good life.

Sheldon and Lyubomirsky (2021) describe developing a few more nuanced models to refine the issues raised by reviews of the sustainable happiness model. These include the hedonic adaptation prevention model (Sheldon & Lyubomirsky, 2012), Lyubomirsky's positive activity model (Lyubomirsky & Layous, 2013), and Sheldon's eudaimonic activity model (Sheldon, 2018). Although we will not delve into the specific details of these models, each one demonstrated in some capacity that individuals could shape their experienced happiness through purposeful efforts. However, Sheldon and Lyubomirsky admit that the resulting effects are usually smaller than what they presumed to be the case from their original 2005 article. More to the point, using double-blind experimental procedures—the desired goal of high-quality psychological research—is rarely possible because volitional happiness studies generally require their participants to have knowledge, understanding, and intentional commitment to well-defined procedures. In other words, participants know what they are doing and why they are doing it.

Sheldon and Lyubomirsky (2021) found that when individuals change their intentional activities by doing something new that requires effort, then they increase the likelihood that a rise in well-being will remain. Such changes differ from the short-lived hedonic boost one encounters when obtaining a new object (e.g., a car, an article of clothing) or windfall (e.g., a higher salary, a promotion). Hedonic adaptation is less likely to occur when a behavior change is based on intrinsic motivation; however, it is more likely to occur when one stable circumstance replaces another (i.e., a "new" car is soon like the "old" car; for specific details, review the hedonic adaptation prevention model; Sheldon & Lyubomirsky, 2012). Furthermore, it can be difficult to "induce" people to do what needs to be done to become happier—dedicated changes in thought and behavior are required, and for many people, they are neither easy to do nor necessarily sustainable across time (Lyubomirsky et al., 2011). Rehabilitation professionals and therapists should keep these facts in mind when recommending activity changes designed to enhance happiness and well-being; people first need to "buy into" the intended changes for benefits to accrue, and in any case, the accompanying effects are apt to be small ones (White et al., 2019). Still, as Sheldon and Lyubomirsky (2021) suggest,

> It might be more accurate to say that people have a *range* of potential well-being rather than a set *point* of well-being. Of course, any such range has a central tendency. A key point of our research has been to show that regression back towards one's prior central tendency might be forestalled, perhaps in the long-term, as a function of one's life choices and behavioral activities. (p. 148, italics in original)

CHOICES, MOTIVATED ACTIONS, ASSETS AND DISABILITY

> If we are right in our view and happiness is assumed to be acting well, the active life will be the best.
>
> —Aristotle (1984, p. 1325b)

Earlier in this chapter, we reviewed the positive psychology literature's recommendations for living a good life, which entail seeking positive connections with others, creating or maintaining positive personal qualities, and exercising life regulation qualities (see also Dunn & Brody, 2008). Following Sheldon and Lyubomirsky (2021), as well as Aristotle, enhanced well-being or happiness (i.e., the good life) can be had by making motivated choices that lead to behaviors that can capitalize on assets. Although the increase in positive feelings may be modest, with ongoing effort, the affective change may remain stable.

Table 6.4 lists some example behaviors in each of the three categories based on people's assets living with or following disability. These are meant to be suggestions, as readers, whether lay or professional, should generate other entries. Naturally, the nature and extent of a person's disability might influence whether an existing entry within a category can apply (Dunn & Brody, 2008). Furthermore, neither disabled persons nor their therapists or family members should seek to enact all the asset entries listed in Table 6.4; rather, judicious care should be taken to select those (or others) that already are or can be acquired assets that complement disabled individuals' interests, abilities, and personalities.

TABLE 6.4

Example Behaviors Linked to Existing or Acquirable Assets that Promote the Good Life with Disability

Connections to other people
Socializing with others
Social comparisons
Helping other people
Positive personal qualities
Finding meaning
Expressing gratitude
Enjoying humor or being humorous
Savoring
Life regulation qualities
Exercise and creature comforts
Finding flow
Special pleasures and self-rewards
Giving back by being generative

Source: Adapted from Dunn and Brody (2008, Table 3, p. 417)

Connections to Others

Close relationships with other people matter a great deal; we are indeed social creatures. Establishing and maintaining close connections, whether with family or friends or both, is important to living well. Making friends and spending quality time with them *socializing* (see Table 6.4), as well as joining groups and networks, is beneficial (Lyubomirsky et al., 2005). Diener and Seligman (2002) found that the number, quality, and regularity of friendly relationships is quite favorable to our well-being. *Social comparison*, a ubiquitous process, allows people to compare their standing on any number of dimensions with that of others (see Table 6.4). When we view someone as being worse off than ourselves, positive self-perceptions often occur whereby we are grateful regarding how our situation differs from the other's (Lockwood, 2002). Identifying with and emulating the acts of others who are doing well despite some setback or problem in order to become like them—what is known as an upward social comparison—can also be a source of motivation to act (Taylor & Lobel, 1989). Finally, *helping other people*, whether directly (e.g., suggesting, advising) or indirectly (e.g., donating) is a simple way to enhance one's mood in a positive direction (e.g., Isen & Levin, 1972; see Table 6.4). The need and desire for meaningful social connection among disabled people should encourage them to look for opportunities to be friendly or to become a friend, just as expressing interest in others usually leads to mutual exchanges that are beneficial.

Positive Personal Qualities

Some of our traits may be genetic in origin, some are learned through observation and experience, and still others can be acquired (recall the VIA Classification of Strengths mentioned earlier in this chapter). Following the onset of disability, several positive personal qualities can be called upon. Some individuals will want to reevaluate their disability by *finding meaning* (ideally, positive aspects) in it (see Table 6.4). Recall that in Chapter 5, found positive meaning was discussed via attributions made by a group of individuals who experienced amputations (see Dunn, 1996). Other people will be able to consciously *express gratitude* for their circumstances despite having a disability (see Table 6.4). Counting one's blessings or the positive aspects of one's life can promote connections to others, prolong positive emotions, slow hedonic adjustment to good events (e.g., Larsen & Prizmic, 2008), and over time, can enhance mood, coping processes, and even lead to self-disclosed health gains (Emmons & McCullough, 2003). *Appreciating humor or being able to express it,* too, can be a positive personal quality (see Table 6.4). Humor can draw people together, leading to positive social encounters, while also helping to adjust to the ups and downs of daily living (e.g., Vaillant, 1995), including perhaps the consequences of disability. Humor is also an effective antidote to stress (e.g., Taylor et al., 2000) and can be a helpful way to cope with and adapt to disability (Burkhead et al., 1996; see also, Marini, 1992). Self-deprecating humor is usually believed to be beneficial, much more so than that aimed at highlighting the pratfalls or plights of others (Dunn & Brody, 2008). Taking time to appreciate daily events and experiences by *savoring* them can also regulate positive emotions in constructive ways (e.g., Bryan & Veroff, 2007; Kurtz, 2018). To savor is to create an exchange between the person and the environment; thoughtfully enjoying a positive experience for its own sake (e.g., listening to music, watching a sunrise) can serve as foil when negative events or feelings emerge.

Life Regulation Qualities

Can setting and meeting goals in daily life enable disabled individuals to have a sense of control? Goal setting and regulation can have additional benefits, such as maintaining health, well-being, and self-control. Getting regular exercise is often identified as way to achieve a healthy life, so perhaps it can also lead to a good life.

Besides benefiting health, regular and moderate *exercise* is a means to maintaining a positive mood and feeling increased energy (see Table 6.4; e.g., Thayer, 2001). Disabled people's perceptions of their ability to exercise should be examined carefully, ensuring that no restrictions on activities exist (i.e., self-grooming, household responsibilities), as they can point to depressive symptoms when accomplishing them is a challenge or even not possible (e.g., Williamson, 1998). Determining the best level of physical exertion that can be expected and performed following a disabling event will be important. Seeking *creature comforts* or actions that promote relaxation and renewal are also important, such as eating, occasionally napping, meditating, or just sitting in silence (see Table 6.4).

Being fully involved in the present moment when doing something is intrinsically rewarding and challenging; otherwise known as *finding flow* (e.g., Csikszentmihalyi, 1997), this is also beneficial (see Table 6.4). These forms of "optimal experience" help individuals become less time- and self-focused so they can engage in pursuits that balance challenge and skill. Such activities include doing creative work, enjoying aesthetic events or hobbies, writing, and playing sports, among many other options (Nakamura & Csikszentmihalyi, 2002). Disabled persons could again pursue interests that trigger flow or search for new ones if previous activities are no longer doable.

Disability can often reveal *special pleasures and self-rewards* (see Table 6.4), or as McBryde Johnson (2005) claimed, some actions "are so bound up with our disabilities that we wouldn't experience them, or wouldn't experience them without our disabilities" (p. 254). Such actions might include learning to speak American Sign Language (ASL) as a socio-political act or racing down a street using a power-wheelchair. Regarding self-rewards, one might have a special treat (e.g., a rich dessert, a special coffee drink) on occasion rather than regularly (e.g., Dunn & Norton, 2014) or even spend time mentally anticipating the pleasures associated with an enjoyable future event (e.g., a trip, a concert; Van Boven & Ashworth, 2007). Such life-regulation efforts represent an effective way to benefit from positive affect and to ward off negative emotions (e.g., Tugade & Fredrickson, 2004).

Finally, life regulation can be achieved by *giving back by being generative* (see Table 6.4). Part of giving back is taking part in the life of a community to positively affect others (e.g., Putnam, 2001). Although this is a form of being helpful, it is more about sharing something tied to oneself (i.e., skills, experiences, knowledge)—being generative (Erikson, 1950, 1986)—that forges meaningful links with others. One can be a mentor or a resource for others, typically younger individuals. An older disabled person could, for example, counsel a recently disabled person concerning what to expect based on the former's own experience. Greater generativity is linked to higher levels of well-being (e.g., Ackerman et al., 2000), which could be associated with perceived commitment (i.e., dealing with adverse circumstances by becoming empathetic). Following Erikson's lead, generative giving aids others but also benefits the self, notably where individual growth and identity matter.

Assets Matter

A focus on people's assets—existing or potential—suggests that a good life following disability is an accessible life. Or, put another way, happiness and well-being are not precluded by congenital or acquired disabilities. Similarly, status values must be replaced by asset values. Disabled individuals, their families and friends, and rehabilitation providers can work together to leverage positive personal qualities to create positive futures.

Precis and Prospects

Psychological assets, the fourth foundational principle, promote the view that disabled persons have or can acquire personal or psychological qualities that enhance behavior and daily life with a disability. Adjustment to disability is possible when assets (or asset values) do not become sources of comparison (or status values) with what was but is no longer. Assets come in a wide variety of forms, so that they are real, perceived, possible, personal, hidden, obvious, or acquirable. The incidence of disability can change or eliminate an asset; yet subsequent effort can restore it or cultivate a new asset. Assets can promote a good life with disability—that is, they can serve as qualities that enhance happiness and well-being, such as forming positive connections with others, creating positive personal qualities, and regulating daily life. Understanding what demographic and other factors are associated (or not) with particular assets can shape people's choices and behaviors following disability onset and into the future. In Chapter 7, we will explore the self-perception of people's bodily states. The idea of perception is key, as people's expectations sometimes govern given bodily states (such as pain or fatigue) but not their actual sensations. In other words, addressing ways to change attitudes and expectations, as well as environments, can alter perception in constructive ways.

THOUGHT QUESTIONS

1. How do status or comparative values differ from asset values? Why do the differences between these terms matter in the case of disability?

2. What is an example of an asset that a disabled person might already have or could relearn or even develop for the first time?
3. Can any disabled person develop an asset or assets?
4. How can the Values in Action (VIA) Classification of Strengths assess the presence of or potential for assets following a disabling event? How do these strengths, virtues, and values likely differ from personality traits?
5. What is the good life? What do you think constitutes the good life following the onset of disability?
6. What factors or variables do and do not predict (in correlational terms) the good life, happiness, or well-being?
7. How can intentional action serve as assets or constructively channel assets for people with disabilities? What are some concrete things they can do to potentially enhance their happiness and well-being, and promote the good life?

7 Principle 5

SELF-PERCEPTION OF BODILY STATES

Foundational Principle 5: Self-Perception of Bodily States

The experience of bodily states (e.g., pain, fatigue, distress) is based on people's perceptions of the phenomena, not exclusively on the actual sensations. Changing attitudes, expectations, or environmental conditions can constructively alter perceptions.

> The significance of a disability is affected by the person's feelings about the self and his or her situation.
>
> —Beatrice A. Wright (1983, p. xii, italics in original)

> It may well turn out that the understanding of experience is the fundamental requirement for the understanding of human beings.
>
> —Daniel M. Wegner & Daniel T. Gilbert (2000, p. 9)

Although psychology, sociology, and even philosophy define the self in many, often complex, ways, most people possess a basic or working understanding of what the self is, even when a clear definition is elusive (Baumeister & Bushman, 2014). The self can be defined as our essence that makes us distinct from others or, more simply, the innate sense of who we are. It can also be the object of our inward focus (i.e., introspection) or even the more outward-looking, public social roles we inhabit

On the Foundational Principles of Rehabilitation Psychology. Dana S. Dunn, Oxford University Press.
 DOI: 10.1093/9780197785188.003.0007

and display. The self is the totality of the individual, including thoughts, feelings, action, agency, and experiential history (APA, 2024a). Of course, there are many other possible definitions as well as theories of the self. We need to be somewhat selective.

A main theory in social psychology—*self-perception theory*—posits that individuals sometimes observe their own behavior to infer their thoughts and feelings—that is, to know themselves (e.g., Bem, 1967, 1972; see also, Nisbett & Valins, 1972). In other words, like someone watching us, we, too, look to see what we are doing and then draw conclusions about what we are like from our own actions. Sometimes, then, the aforementioned introspective processes or self-reflection fails us (e.g., Nisbett & Wilson, 1977; Wilson, 2002), and we are not sure how we think or feel about something. When we don't know ourselves in some capacity, we often see what we do (or have done) to obtain an answer.

Whether we look inward or outward, however, we are trying to understand and make sense of our subjective experiences—our thoughts and feelings—as a person at a moment in time (Wegner & Gilbert, 2000). Why does this matter in the context of disability? Because how disabled people subjectively experience their conditions has an influence on how well they navigate the rehabilitation process and whether they adjust and accept their disabilities (recall Chapter 5). Rehabilitation practitioners are well aware that how people experience some bodily states, such as pain or fatigue, is based on their insider self-perceptions, not only the actual felt sensations, but also on the presumed attitudes of outsiders (e.g., Fordyce 1976). In social psychology, attribution theory research clearly demonstrates that people do not see their realities from a veridical perspective (recall Chapter 3). Rather, their perceptions of reality (including the presumed reality of others) are tempered or even biased by expectations (their own and those of others), stereotypes, and the recall of past experiences (e.g., Fiske & Taylor, 2014; Pronin et al., 2004).

Indeed, as we learned earlier, Wilson (2022) argues that social psychology is founded on the *construal principle*, so that understanding and predicting human behavior requires researchers to know people's proximate (current) construals of themselves and their environment. Social construals are linked to people's environments and social norms, and if shaped into a constructive intervention, these self-explanations can be used to change human behavior in a favorable direction (e.g., Walton & Wilson, 2018; Wilson, 2011). By extension, for rehabilitation psychologists and their allies to supportively work with people with disabilities, appreciating how they see themselves and their circumstances—including their experienced bodily states and physique—will have an important influence on their quality of life and outlooks following a disabling event.

Thus, in this chapter, we will explore how the fifth foundational principle can inform theory and practice. We begin by discussing somatopsychology and its influence on disabled people's self-perceptions.

Somatopsychology and Self-Perception

> The somatopsychological relation involves social-psychological factors, that is, factors that underlie the way disability as a value loss is perceived and reacted to by other people, as well as the self. Actually, much of the psychology of the individual requires social-psychological understanding, since the way in which one feels and behaves about many things depends in greater or lesser measure upon one's relationship with other persons.
>
> —Beatrice A. Wright (1983, p. 6)

The *somatopsychological relation*, as defined by Barker et al. (1953), examines how variations in physique (i.e., the build, shape, and/or form of the body) influence an individual's self-image, their social exchanges with others, and the activities and behaviors they choose or decline to pursue (see also Barker, 1947; Wright, 1983). Barker and colleagues observed that

> [the] relation between physique and behavior arises because the body is a tool with physical properties that make it possible for a person to engage in some activities and not others. The definition of what activities are possible for a particular physique may be arbitrarily imposed by authority . . . or it may be developed through trial and error. (1953, p. 3)

Physical disability generally entails some form of altered physique, whether congenital or acquired. A body part or parts might be missing or appear in an altered form or forms, or a limb or limbs may function differently or not at all. A person's body may also be intact where outward appearance is concerned, but movement through space may be done differently, that is, in an unaccustomed manner or with some type of aid (e.g., a cane, a walker, a wheelchair, a service animal). Adopting a somewhat broader perspective, disabilities that are not viewed as typically physical in nature (e.g., sensory, intellectual, psychiatric, chronic health conditions as disabilities) or are "hidden" can also be understood through a similar lens: Some quality or qualities are manifest that render the individual distinct and different (recall the discussion of the WHO model in Chapter 1). Such qualities can affect how the person thinks about themselves and their abilities and behavioral choices, as well as how others (i.e., outsiders) perceive their abilities, actions, and options.

Clearly, the person-environment relation and its implications are relevant to somatopsychology (recall Chapter 3), yet the latter remains, as Dunn (2015) wrote, "more important than any psychosomatic connection of an organic or physical disorder to the individual's psychology" (p. 27). Wright (1983) describes an everyday example of the somatopsychological problem many people with acquired disabilities face. The key here is to appreciate the fact that such problems can appear to be personal ones on initial appraisal but are usually found to have a profoundly social basis. Imagine an individual who has a recently acquired disability is found to be struggling with some basic routines of daily life, such as getting dressed and eating meals. The person can perform these behaviors only with great difficulty, and thus there is a difference between what can be done and the required tasks that need to be accomplished. Slipping on slacks, putting on socks, tying shoelaces, and using a knife, fork, and spoon, while familiar, are suddenly challenges to perform. There is an overlooked social element here—the expectations for how one must dress, the types and design of the clothes to be worn, that food must be consumed in a certain manner; these are "*ways of behavior prescribed by society*" and as such represent subtle but powerful social psychological forces (italics are Wright's [1983]). Alternate ways to dress and eat could be found, just as clothes and dining implements can be redesigned to be more accessible and useful; these are environmental changes that can be made to fit a person's particular needs, but only if effort in this direction is initiated.

Too often, established routine mired in sociocultural tradition dictates choice and action. This analysis matters because newly disabled individuals may feel compelled to perform activities in accustomed ways to be "like everyone else," a desire to fit in or to return to what once was, which is often counterproductive and personally devaluing, to use Wright's (1983) term. As we discussed in Chapter 6, comparative values can be problematic, and new asset values, recently acquired assets, and ways of doing things can be identified and learned.

Let's consider another hypothetical but possible example. A solider lost his left hand and much of his left arm (above the elbow) in a roadside bombing in Afghanistan. He is a dedicated cyclist who enjoyed competitive racing. Following the trauma, he underwent extensive rehabilitation and obtained a prosthetic arm and hand, which he learned to use. He wanted to ride again, so he was not concerned with the plastic and metallic nature of the prostheses, nor did he care much about the attention and curiosity they might create in the minds of others when he was learning to cycle again. He was conscious that outsiders might objectify him or offer unsolicited and unwanted "admiration," but he deemed those risks acceptable to regain the joy he felt when biking.

Another soldier with a similar loss or someone who lost an arm in an industrial accident might decline the chance to cycle again with a prosthetic limb precisely because of worry about his altered physique. Perhaps riding a bike and racing will be different now, just as people (including some family and friends, as well as strangers) may stare and ask questions or remain silent, awkward, and surprised at his appearance. These concerns—which are based on his social psychological sense of self and others—are tied to his changed physique and presumed social opinion, thereby trumping his wish to cycle again. In both cases, the protagonists' psychosocial adjustments to their similar circumstances were not solely dependent on the disability itself; rather, the individuals and their perceived physical, social, and psychological environments were affected by their somatopsychology.

INFERRING PAIN

As noted earlier, perceived pain may only partially be due to pain-producing stimuli. Consider the consequences of self-observation serving as a source of pain perception. How accurate is it? Bandler et al. (1968) explored the hypothesis that people's perception of a stimulus as being uncomfortable or painful is at least in part inferred from their own observation of their responses to that stimulus. College-aged participants observed themselves either escaping from or enduring a series of electric shocks, all of which had the same physical intensity. As the investigators predicted, the participants rated the discomfort produced by the shocks to be greater in the "escape" condition than in the "no-escape" condition. As Bandler et al. argued,

> An affirmative reply to the question, "Was the last electric shock uncomfortable?," may be functionally equivalent to the individual's (or an outside observer's) saying, "It must have been; I (he) attempted to escape it as quickly as possible." In other words, an individual's behavioral response to an aversive stimulus, often treated as a dependent variable in pain research, may serve as an independent variable and partially control his perception of the stimulus as uncomfortable or painful. (p. 205)

A review of the participants' galvanic skin responses (i.e., the change in the electrical resistance of the skin caused by emotional stress) indicated that the actual physiological arousal did not act as the basis for their discomfort ratings. Instead, the participants inferred higher levels of pain by observing their own responses to the shocks (which lasted for precisely the same duration in both conditions).

Within the rehabilitation psychology community, Wilbert Fordyce (1976) pioneered the behavioral assessment and treatment of chronic pain patients by relying on understanding how patients viewed and reacted to their own pain responses. His work was a reaction to the "either-or" perspective that was prevalent in pain research: Either the patient's pain was real or it was psychogenic (i.e., pain associated with psychological rather than physical factors) in origin. Instead, Fordyce turned the focus to critically explore specific social and environmental influences on both the clients' pain behaviors and well behaviors, so that increases in the latter and decreases in the former were sought. He and his colleagues applied operant-based methods to help people with their management of chronic pain.

People's perceptions and, in turn, their behaviors were found to be malleable, so they could be influenced or altered in adaptive or maladaptive directions on the basis of attitudes (their own and those of observers, including health care professionals), expectations (their own or those offered by family, friends, and medical team members), and environmental reinforcement (physical, social, and psychological). Based on these insights, rehabilitation practitioners and researchers try to shape clients' perceptions in positive ways to promote psychosocial adjustment to pain and disability, while also seeking a beneficial person-environment relation that focuses on their individual worth (for contemporary views of Fordyce's classic work, see Main et al., 2015).

Self-Esteem and Body Image

Appearances—how one sees oneself and how we believe others see us—matter a great deal. Although personal preference plays a role, the aesthetics of beauty and attractiveness are largely culturally and socially dictated. These influences, which are inescapable due to social media and advertising, affect self-image, one's sense of sexual desirability, and inevitably, self-esteem. As a psychological construct, self-esteem entails a person's overall assessment of their worth as a person, and it is partially dependent on people's social self-image and their physical self-image (e.g., Shavelson et al., 1976).

Disability onset can sometimes alter a person's physical appearance. Depending on where and how the person's body is changed, societal expectations for body image and the attitudes one has toward one's physical sense of self may decrease, thereby adversely affecting self-esteem (Graf & Glover, 2024). When a person's self-esteem is low, they have less confidence and are less willing to pursue social activities or relationships with other people. Less opportunity for socializing can lead to isolation and a lower quality of life, so that rejection by others seems certain. The presence of a physical anomaly or anomalies can heighten concerns about being objectified or even laughed at as well as creating feelings of deviance and stigma (recall Chapter 1). Facial disfigurement poses an even greater challenge, as its link to self-image and identity is a distinct one that stands out from the rest of the physical body. Callahan (2004), who examined such disfigurement among individuals with head and neck cancer, pointed to "profound psychological trauma" (p. 73) linked to people's reduced sense of self and body integrity.

Indeed, Callahan (2004) suggested that each part of the body has some symbolic meaning beyond its functional use. Hands can represent creativity and arms suggest strength, just as legs entail vitality, volition, and speed. The genitalia and reproductive organs represent intimacy, pleasure, and procreative potential. Age and sex can also make a difference where visible differences are concerned, as adolescents and younger adults express greater levels of concern regarding appearance than middle-aged and older individuals, just as women do over men (Graf & Glover, 2024).

Physical appearance, then, can have profound consequences for psychosocial adjustment and adaptation. Rehabilitation psychologists cannot ignore this fact, as how affected persons feel about themselves is linked not only to social interaction (or the lack thereof) but also to depression, anxiety, shame, and the social avoidance of other people. Social support and interaction can promote some adjustment to disfigurement (Kleve et al., 2002). Pride in disability and ties to the disability community can also mediate associations between stigmatization and lower self-esteem, thereby affording some safeguards for the self and ego (Bogart et al., 2018 and related discussions of disability identity in Chapter 5). In other words, changing one's values can provide a means to maintain positive self-regard.

VALUES REVISITED

Where dealing with self-esteem and body image issues is concerned, it should be clear that disabled persons should be counseled away from using comparative values and instead learn to focus on new or acquirable asset values (recall Chapter 6). Wright (1983; see also Marini & Villarreal, 2024) suggested three other forms of value change that can aid people with disabilities. They are:

Enlarging the Scope of Their Values

The goal here is for affected individuals to stop pursuing values or predisability activities that they no longer can reliably perform due to physique alterations and elect to expand their list of interests and activities to align with their new capabilities, as well as asset values and assets. For example, a now-disabled athlete could engage in online gaming in place of the physical versions that were once sought. The goal is to focus on one's current and future potential rather than reviewing or even ruminating over lost or dormant abilities.

Subordination of One's Physique

Here, the individual engages in cognitively reframing what individual qualities or self-related aspects matter in lieu of a physical persona. Thus, a person who once focused on physical appearance and related qualities (e.g., athleticism) will need to redefine the importance of nonphysical attributes, such as intelligence, humor, or key personality traits, among other possibilities. In effect, emphasis on the body shifts to an emphasis on the mind or character, which represents a different but nonetheless important and social facet of the self.

Containment of Disability Effects

Individuals with acquired disabilities should not allow their disability to "spread" to other parts of their being (recall the related discussion in Chapter 4). The aftermath of a stroke may lead to aphasia, for example, manifesting itself as slower speech production. The affected person needs to make clear to outsiders that their memory and intellect remain unaffected. Similarly, disabled people must not allow strangers to ask their nondisabled family members or companions about their preferences (e.g., when ordering a meal in a restaurant, selecting a purchase in a store, choosing where to sit in a concert); they must learn to assert themselves and establish their autonomy despite their disability and the sometimes-infantilizing behavior of intrusive outsiders. As new asset values and assets replace old ones, disabled individuals can navigate their life domains and seek well-being by following how they feel (or adjusting their feelings in favorable directions).

Life Domains and Well-Being: How People Feel

Fleming, Umucu, and Phillips (2024) identified ways to promote opportunity and function within life domains valued by people with disabilities and chronic illnesses. They argue that both insiders and outsiders share positive views regarding the importance of these life domains; however, insiders often face structural and psychological barriers—such as inaccessible venues, being marginalized, or simple social exclusion—that limit their ability to be satisfied, let alone being able to flourish. Valued roles, autonomy and choice, and physical and mental health will be briefly considered. Please note that each one can influence and is, in turn, affected by the somatopsychological issues experienced by disabled individuals.

VALUED SOCIAL ROLES

Although people inhabit a variety of social roles across their lives (e.g., spouse, parent, neighbor, friend, coworker), some roles appear to be more important than others where well-being is concerned. In the United States, what you do for a living—variously referred to as occupation, career, or job—has a profound effect on one's social standing and self-esteem. Increasingly, disability is a concern for the workplace as well as for people with disabilities (Cheng et al., 2019). The presence of a disability sometimes compromises employability for a variety of reasons, including the need for supports or workplace accommodations, training or educational issues, as well as employment discrimination due to ableism (Dunn, 2015; Fleming et al., 2024). For these and other reasons, disabled persons can be underemployed (i.e., holding a place in the workforce for which they are overqualified and often underpaid) or unemployed. Being unemployed has very negative consequences for anyone, disabled or not, as it reduces well-being, happiness, self-confidence, and the overall sense of self (Weiten et al., 2024; recall unemployment as one of the variables that negatively influenced the good life in Chapter 6). Mental and physical health, too, can be undermined by a lack of consequential employment (Wanberg, 2012).

Remedies to alleviate employment issues for people with disabilities remain a challenge. To some degree, other valued social roles may be able to compensate for one's work status. Still, as a social psychological factor in American life, what one does for a living is significant, as it is tied to income, social class, social status, being a provider for the family, self-image, and so on. Rehabilitation counselors should keep employment and career issues in mind when working with their clients, especially those who are recently disabled. The loss of a desirable career can represent a profound change to a valued social role as well an important part of a person's identity.

AUTONOMY AND CHOICE: SELF-DETERMINATION

Humans are very social beings, yet at times they prefer to act alone and independently. Being autonomous means that you can make your own decisions rather than being told what to do by some other person or entity. Autonomy is a strong human need, one that also affects well-being (Deci & Ryan, 2000). Disability need not decrease perceived autonomy, though some persons with disabilities do encounter environmental or attitudinal barriers (recall Chapter 3). Some rely on ongoing assistance, while others may receive overprotection from family and friends. The latter phenomenon is especially salient among individuals with intellectual or developmental disabilities, as well as persistent mental illness (Fleming et al., 2024). These groups often require some form of guardianship or care that controls or even inhibits their ability to run their own lives and ongoing situations (Kohn et al., 2013). Research clearly demonstrates that self-determination, independence, and self-control enhance people's quality of life (Wehmeyer, 2019). In fact, autonomy-supportive interventions demonstrate that instruction coupled with learning opportunities, for example, can help adolescents with disabilities gain skills and beliefs that allow them to develop into causal agents in their own lives—that is, they can become self-determined adults.

PHYSICAL AND MENTAL HEALTH MATTERS

Disabled people are much more likely to be diagnosed with poor health than are nondisabled people. Their life spans tend to be shorter than their nondisabled counterparts, and they frequently experience medical complications and hospitalizations, as well as sicknesses that are preventable (Fleming et al., 2024). These factors also point to psychological consequences, such as depression and anxiety. Disabled individuals are also more likely to lead sedentary existences, to smoke, and to be unhealthily overweight, factors that are often linked with diabetes and heart disease (Lollar et al., 2021). The consequences of their conditions lead disability to be a serious public health issue. There are a variety of approaches to health and wellness designed to combat the comorbidities posed by disability and other chronic health conditions. Self-management of healthy behaviors among disabled individuals is linked with well-being, just as mobility-designed interventions can ameliorate physical (and psychological) changes among older disabled persons, thereby maintaining their quality of life (Groessl et al., 2019; Ravesloot et al., 2016). Dealing with such challenges requires acceptance of bodily or physique-related realities, as well as some self-image realignment and an expansion of values (e.g., health is more important than pleasurable but ultimately unhealthy habits, like smoking, excess consumption of alcohol, recreational drugs, and the like).

FEELINGS

Wright (1983) advocated that a client's feelings and point of view are central to rehabilitation efforts. Affirmation of the client's dignity and lived experience can enhance the effectiveness of professional interventions or therapeutic guidance. Emotional support—being understood, listened to, and involved in a genuine therapeutic alliance—can advance positive changes in cognition and behavior. Regarding the role of feelings or affect, Fordyce (1971) argued,

> Information about and understanding of the individual's feelings can facilitate behavioral approaches by helping to identify how the person discriminates stimulus situations and by indicating what environmental events are likely to be reinforcing or nonreinforcing to him. In addition, most people identify effective or important attention from others with the other person being interested in and responsive to expressions of one's own feelings. The development of an effective treatment relationship with a client or patient... can be enhanced considerably by the professional's awareness of his client's (verbal or nonverbal feelings). What is suggested here is that a more expeditious way to help the disabled person is to focus on helping him to change his behavior. It is quite possible that feelings will follow rather than lead these behavior changes. (pp. 77–78)

Disability-Affirmative Therapy

Much of this chapter is focused on helping insiders navigate new somatopsychological relations in their daily lives. Doing so often involves a focus on behavior change as well as changes in values and recognition of new or obtainable assets. Yet more may be needed where culturally competent intervention is concerned, as many psychologists, though well-intentioned, lack sufficient knowledge and experience working with clients with disabilities (Andrews, 2020; Olkin, 2017). To address these and related concerns, Olkin (2007, 2017; see also 1999) advocated establishing a *disability-affirmative therapy* (DAT), which outlined a template for applying psychotherapeutic principles to work with disabled persons that is grounded in a biopsychosocial view of disability (e.g., Dunn, 2015).

There are two main components to DAT. The first entails areas of exploration for disabled clients and their families. The nine areas are a developmental history, current disability status, disability models, additional demographic and cultural identities (i.e., intersectional factors), disability culture and community, social interaction, understanding microaggressions, emotional management, and relational intimacy. Reflecting on issues and experiences in these areas prepares the client for beginning the actual therapy.

The second component entails a therapeutic stance that Olkin (2017) created by consulting various other therapeutic approaches (e.g., gay affirmative therapy). DAT is designed to be more of a framework for understanding clients than a specific technique. This framework presumes that the presence of a disability does not necessarily entail pathology but can provide values and inherent meaning to their ongoing experiences. Olkin recommends that disabled individuals should affirm a disability identity by finding positive disabled role models and mentors, getting involved with the disability community, and working to positively reframe any stigmatizing traits, qualities long associated with disability studies research (e.g., Olkin & Pledger, 2003). By seeking out these social-communal resources and exploring available assistive technologies (e.g., for mobility, communication, and sensory issues), clients can improve their daily lives. Part of exploring such shared experiences entails reflecting frankly on encountered microaggressions during the therapeutic process. By doing so, clients can come to better understand their emotional reactions and develop effective responses for future social exchanges.

Clearly, DAT seems to be a constructive way to help disabled persons, especially newly disabled ones, to navigate, understand, and accept their experiences. This framework is also a way to potentially avoid the problems associated with internalized ableism (see Nario-Redmond, 2020). Yet to date, there is no solid empirical evidence to support the scope and claims underlying DAT, a point made by Olkin (2017). There is still a paucity of evidence-based treatments for people with disabilities. DAT appears to be a compelling approach, but research verifying its effectives remains to be conducted. Still, rehabilitation and allied professionals would do well to familiarize themselves with its tenets to better work with clients who are coming to terms with their somatopsychological relations and feelings.

Precis and Prospects

This chapter explored how to understand, interpret, and build on subjective states following the onset of disability. At times, disabled persons look to their situations or social circumstances to explain their feelings and sensations, which means pain, fatigue, distress, anxiety, and the like can be malleable to therapeutic intervention. This self-perception can then be a tool for the rehabilitation therapist or practitioner. Somatopsychology entails the ways physique affects self and other relations, which means it is highly influenced by the first foundational principle, the person-environment relation. Self-esteem, too, is tied to body image, and views on the latter may encourage an audit and possible changes of values. How people feel about their subjective experience matters a great deal and allows for the potential use of DAT. In the next chapter, we will build on the subjective elements of somatopsychology to consider foundational principle 6, the importance of maintaining disabled people's sense of human dignity regardless of the nature or extent of their disabilities or other chronic health conditions.

THOUGHT QUESTIONS

1. Why is subjective human experience an important factor where understanding people's bodily states is concerned? How does *self-perception theory* relate to this issue?
2. What is *somatopsychology*? What is the *somatopsychological relation*?
3. How do social psychological factors, like one's culture, potentially affect construal of disability as well as behavioral adaptation or change?
4. How can inferred pain or other sensations be influenced (or informed) by social psychological factors?
5. How is self-esteem tied to *physique*? How can changes in values retain or bolster positive self-regard? How do life domains affect well-being and feelings?
6. What is *disability-affirmative therapy* (DAT)? Why does it currently remain an unproven approach to help people with disabilities?

8 Principle 6

THE IMPORTANCE OF HUMAN DIGNITY

Foundational Principle 6: The Importance of Human Dignity

Regardless of the source or severity of a disability or chronic health condition, all people deserve respect and encouragement and to be treated with dignity.

> A person is entitled to the enrichment of life and the development of his or her abilities, whether these be great or small and whether the person has a long or short time to live. The person must not be led to devaluate the self or to give up hope. The person is not to remain neglected and deprived.
>
> —Beatrice A. Wright (1983, p. xi)

> Disability is only one aspect, and often a very minor aspect, of a *person*. We should always attend primarily to the person.
>
> —Harold E. Yuker (1988, p. xiv, italics in original)

> An essential core-concept of human dignity is that a person is not an object, not a thing.
>
> —Beatrice A. Wright (1987, p. 12)

What do we mean by *human dignity*? Why does human dignity matter in general as well as in the specific context of disability and chronic illness? These questions

On the Foundational Principles of Rehabilitation Psychology. Dana S. Dunn, Oxford University Press.
 DOI: 10.1093/9780197785188.003.0008

are the focus of this chapter, though we will view them through the lens of the sixth foundational principle.

Human dignity entails believing that every person possesses a special quality that is linked to their humanity—that is, the state of being human. This quality is independent of one's gender, race or ethnicity, religion, abilities or lack thereof, or any other demographic or social grouping variable (recall Chapter 2). Human dignity also entails the fact that every person is equal to all other people and has an inherent and undisputable value like every other person. All people deserve to be respected for their own sake, just as they must be treated in an ethical and moral manner.

The foundation of this perspective is based in the Enlightenment, an intellectual and cultural movement in 17th- and 18th-century Europe in which ideas about nature, reason, humanity, and God became synthesized into a worldview that spread widely (e.g., Gay, 1995, 1996). Among the goals of this rational view of humanity were the creation of knowledge, the importance of freedom, and the pursuit of individual happiness. In the present day, Enlightenment values underlie our notions of identity, citizenship, equality, and the right to privacy, as well as the right to education, employment, and healthcare, among other factors.

Disability, Values, and Dignity

> The hard reality is this: Society in every nation is still infected by the ancient assumption that people with disabilities are less than fully human and therefore, are not fully eligible for the opportunities which are available to other people as a matter of right.
>
> —Justin Dart (1992)

Concern about the importance of values resonates through the foundational principles (e.g., Dunn et al., 2016), the spirit and goals of the Americans with Disabilities Act (1990), and Wright's (1983) value-laden beliefs and principles. For example, point 1 of the latter is the precursor to foundational principle 6: "*Every individual needs respect and encouragement; the presence of a disability, no matter how severe, does not alter these fundamental rights*" (p. xi, italics in original). Wright specifically claimed that any person deserves an enriched life and the cultivation of their abilities (whether great or small), irrespective of whether that person's life span will be long or short. No one has the right to eliminate hope in the person, to encourage their self-devaluation, or to neglect or deprive the person in any way. Nor should the person ever be treated as an object or, in contemporary parlance, in an ableist manner.

Wright (1983) was opposed to permitting biases that rendered the members of some groups more deserving than others (Andrews et al., 2021), an issue we will revisit in Chapter 9. As Wright put it, "Life, increased mobility, and better communication skills are as important to a 72-year-old as to a 12-year-old, . . . to a black person as to a white person, to a poor person as to a rich person (p. xi)." Where limited resources are concerned, human worth and accompanying dignity must be considered when any allocation decisions are made.

Point 16 in the value-laden beliefs and principles is that "*people with disabilities, like all citizens, are entitled to participate in and contribute to the general life of the community*" (Wright, 1983, p. xvi, italics in original). In Wright's view, disabled persons should not be regarded only as consumers; rather, they should be recognized for the skills and talents that make them a resource for the larger community. Additionally, point 16 subtly acknowledges the regrettable history of disability, when individuals were often segregated or "warehoused" in special facilities, institutions, or schools, thereby being denied the experience of mainstream living and the many opportunities afforded to their nondisabled peers (for histories of disabled people's exclusion in the United States and abroad, see Andrews, 2020 and Fox & Marini, 2024). As we have learned, there are still attitudinal and environmental barriers that preclude people with disabilities from full participation where education, employment and underemployment, and income, among other arenas, are concerned.

As evidence for these barriers, Andrews (2020) and Marini (2024) provide examples of prevalent myths and stereotypes about disability that sorely affect the dignity of people with disabilities. These distorted beliefs are often found in various media, our contemporary culture, and societal attitudes (which will be explored in more detail below) and are inherently ableist. Table 8.1 lists some of these myths and stereotypes (and, sadly, readers may think of others that could be included), which are all too familiar and likely to influence the thoughts, feelings, and actions of many nondisabled people when they encounter disabled peers.

Use of the word "person" has been a prominent feature of writing and research on disability since the field of rehabilitation psychology emerged. We will discuss its historical and contextual importance next.

The *Person*: A Brief Digression

Most psychologists are familiar with the word "person" if only because it is frequently evoked in the context of the study of human personality. Within that field, some psychologists have used the word person in particular ways that highlight notions of identity. Others have focused on how persons want to be treated and

TABLE 8.1

Some Prevalent Myths and Stereotypes About Disability that Reduce Human Dignity
Disability is always a tragedy.
People with disabilities are perpetual children (i.e., in need of constant care).
Disabled people are or should be objects of pity.
People with disabilities need to be cured of their conditions.
Disabled people with mental illness are a threat to society.
Some people with disabilities are helpless, sick, asexual, and incompetent.
Disabled people are always seeking special privileges.
Enabling disability access harms businesses financially.
Integrating disabled children reduces resources for nondisabled children.
People with disabilities should really get their needs met through charity.
Disabled people do not have to contribute to society, as they are incapable of doing so.

Source: Adapted from Andrews (2020) and Marini (2024)

understood by others. "Personology" has been proposed as a more precise alternative to "personality," though it has not caught on in the field. Humanistic psychologists who study personality adopt the perspective that to truly understand someone, you must learn that person's view of reality. One of the early humanistically oriented psychologists, Carl Rogers (1902–1987), founded what is known as person-centered (sometimes called client-centered) therapy. Rogers argued that people have a basic need to *actualize* themselves, by which he meant they possess a drive or orientation to maintain and enhance their lives. From this perspective, the goal of people's existence is to satisfy this need—that is, to become self-actualized, to evolve into the best person one can be (which is admittedly a challenge to define clearly and a frequent criticism of the humanistic approach).

What does self-actualization actually entail? In part, it means that one should live in ways that lead to a clear understanding of reality and the self (e.g., Funder, 2024). People who perceive the world accurately (i.e., without distortions tied to various neuroses) and who also accept responsibility for their choices (good and bad) can become *fully functioning persons.* In Rogers's view, such people are happy and not plagued by fears, worries, or self-doubt; they have very low or no neurotic tendencies. They must, however, have experienced *unconditional positive regard* from their role models (e.g., parents, teachers, peers); that is, no matter how they have behaved (within some reasonable boundaries), they always have been accepted and loved for who they are. But if they sense that they are valued by important others if—and only if—they display certain qualities (e.g., being smart, attractive, good, successful, obedient, or whatever), they will develop *conditions of worth* or criteria they feel must be met to continue to receive *conditional positive regard* from those around them who matter.

Conditional positive regard entails agreeing to meet certain expectations to be liked or loved; failing to do so means that important others will withdraw their affection and respect unless and until the desired conditions are met, which is stressful as well as controlling. Meeting and maintaining such conditions can damage self-esteem as well as limit people's choice and freedom to think or act. We have all experienced or even fallen prey to such conditions (e.g., "If I do not maintain a high grade point average, I will fail my family." "My parents have done so much for me. Although I want to become a teacher, I will become the engineer they want.") or seen them experienced by others (e.g., an adult friend who continues to follow parental directives rather than her own desires, a lonely person who spurned a seemingly ideal partner his family did not embrace).

How do these ideas work in Rogers's psychotherapy with clients? Rogerian therapy entails the therapist trying to help a client perceive the client's own feelings and thoughts without the therapist changing them in any way. At the same time, the therapist works to make the client feel respected and valued without regard to what the client might think, say, or do. In other words, this therapeutic process provides the client with insight into themselves while also blocking conditions of worth, thereby (theoretically) enabling the client to become more of a fully functioning person. This approach requires quite a bit of time and patience, and the results are admittedly mixed. If nothing else, however, the notion of client-centered therapy has influenced other approaches to psychotherapy to embrace listening closely and as nonjudgmentally as possible to clients (Funder, 2024).

Rehabilitation practitioners and their allies are not likely to be Rogerians (i.e., loyal followers of Carl Rogers's theory and therapy), yet they do understand the importance of listening intently to their disabled clients' ideas, experiences, and hopes, leveraging them to meet rehabilitative ends. When referring to clients, they may elect to use person-first phrases, such as "person with a disability" or "people with disabilities," thereby emphasizing the person first rather than the disability (but see Dunn & Andrews, 2015; recall also Chapter 2). They also try to understand and accept the clients' views of the realities tied to their disabilities (though they do sometimes try to shape them in constructive directions; recall Chapter 7). To meet a client's needs, the practitioner must know and respect that person as well as the person's construal of disability. Interestingly, Beatrice Wright studied with Rogers for a year during her graduate training, and his clinical perspective informed the compassionate message found in much of her writing about and clinical work with disabled individuals. Indeed, she believed in and advocated for professional obligations that promoted human dignity.

Professional Obligations and Human Dignity

Wright (1987) was particularly interested in advocating for human dignity as it related to rehabilitation counselor-client relationships; in her view, the former should always place the latter's interests above their own. Conceptually, this was the foundation of all ethical standards linked to rehabilitation experiences. Or as Wright explained,

> Being a person and not a thing means that I have feelings and ideas; things don't. I have needs, aspirations, and fears that matter. They are important to me. If I am to be treated like a human being they must not be dismissed or ignored. Without my ideas, my feelings, my needs, my hopes, and my fears, I am nothing—just a thing. But I am not a thing! I am a person, a human being! So listen to me; give weight to my needs and ideas; share with me! (p. 12)

Wright (1987) encouraged rehabilitation counselors to observe four hierarchical principles (where successive principles presumed the acceptance of prior ones). These principles were to be altered only when obvious exceptions emerged—and then only after thoughtful reflection accompanied by clear and justifiable explanation.

1. *Clients and counselors must operate as both a provider and recipient of information.* A chair does not care where it is placed or how it is treated, but clients certainly do. Information—plans for treatment, for example—must be shared and accepted in advance. While this might seem obvious, all too often procedures are imposed on clients with no explanation, which is a form of objectification.
2. *Clients must act as comanagers during rehabilitation.* Clients have both the ability and the right—and in consultation with their therapists—to create and sort through alternatives and to reflect on and respond to all decisions involving their care and welfare.
3. *Clients are entitled to serve as vital members of the team working on their behalf.* Like other team members, clients are also experts because they know things about their conditions that no one else knows so well or intimately. These include what hurts, the nature of their circumstances, their feelings

and worries, and their thoughts and hopes for the future. Moreover, "*ideas that may emerge during the actual team meeting*" (italics are Wright's; p. 12) are crucial for developing and understanding effective rehabilitative plans.

4. *Clients have the right to make choices and to veto decisions made for them.* Wright observed that this right applied whenever it is primarily the client's life that is being affected. Clients may also need encouragement and support to appreciate and embrace their own dignity. Professionals as well as clients may need assistance in accepting their comanagement roles (see Wright, 1983). If not, clients may accept the "sick role" as the appropriate, if regrettable, solution.

Of course, aspects of certain cases may alter or otherwise qualify these boundaries of human dignity. Disabled children, for example, may have less of a say when planning their treatment than will most adults. Individuals with severe mental or intellectual incapacities, too, may not be able to take part in essential decision-making. Finally, prisoners do not share the same rights of self-governance as do others. Yet even so, any changes or justifications must be carefully performed so that administrative convenience, habit, "established" rules, desired speed or efficiencies, or any other preferences do not weaken the four principles and thereby the dignity of the affected individual.

AVOIDING SUBTLE VIOLATIONS OF DIGNITY

Medical communities develop their own cultures, including unwritten but accepted rules and ways of doing things. Wright (1987) remained concerned that even everyday language in these professional settings could undermine client sovereignty and dignity. As we have noted previously, imagine how one doctor might speak to another or to a nurse about a client or patient in passing as "the quad in room 227" or "the stroke in rehab unit 3." Such short communications do convey information, but at the same time they eliminate the personhood of the individuals being discussed—the fact that they are not present does not excuse the objectifying nature of what is said. Is it too difficult to instead say "the man with quadriplegia in room 227" or the "woman who had a stroke in rehab unit 3"? Not at all. So, there is really no place for such medical devaluation of clients. More to the point, if the clients are actively involved in discussions about their care and treatment plans, these sorts of egregious and ableist statements would never, ever be made.

What about the role of expertise? Some readers, notably professionals, may worry that client involvement in discussions and decisions somehow reduces or even undermines the skills of medical staff. It should not do so if they are openminded regarding the potentially helpful and authentic perspectives being offered by clients as comanagers. Wouldn't trained professionals welcome insights from clients that could refine their own rehabilitative and therapeutic techniques? In addition, are there not benefits for clients who perceive the interest of team members as representing emotional involvement and support—that is, an underlying message that the medical staff truly cares (see Leviton, 1973)?

Concerns about beliefs and attitudes held by rehabilitation professionals are not limited to the idea of counselors and clients as comanagers. There is considerable evidence that many healthcare professionals harbor stigmatizing attitudes toward people with disabilities, which represents another source of concern regarding human dignity.

HEALTHCARE PROFESSIONALS' ATTITUDES TOWARD DISABILITY: ANOTHER SOURCE OF CONCERN

Unfortunately, it is rather well-established that the attitudes of some healthcare professionals toward disabled persons are decidedly negative (e.g., Marini, 2024). Before explaining why this occurs, let's define the attitude construct.

An attitude is a hypothetical construct and a global evaluation of an individual, an idea, an object, or an issue that is favorable, unfavorable, or ambivalent (i.e., based on a mix of the prior two reactions) (e.g., Banaji & Heiphetz, 2010; Dunn, 2015; Eagly & Chaiken, 1993). Attitudes are said to have a cognitive component, an affective component, and a behavioral component (e.g., Breckler, 1984). The *cognitive component* represents beliefs and can be based on personal perspectives or facts (e.g., "I believe that disabled people should receive necessary accommodations in the classroom."). Emotion is tied to the *affective component* (e.g., "I am frustrated when nondisabled people request classroom accommodations when they do not need them."). How people respond behaviorally (or expect to do so in the future) is linked to the *behavioral component* (e.g., "Before I grant any accommodations, I will make sure the student completed the necessary paperwork at the Office of Accommodations."). Attitudes are different from *beliefs*, which are either opinions or facts about someone or something (for a detailed discussion of the attitude construct as an essential subject in the social psychology of disability, see Andrews, 2020 and Dunn, 2015).

A recent survey study of 714 US physicians by Iezzoni et al. (2021) discerned some discomforting ableist perspectives. For example, 82.4% of the doctors reported that they believe that individuals with significant disabilities experience a worse quality of life than nondisabled people, a common but prevalent falsehood. Just 40.7% of the same group of doctors were very confident regarding their own abilities to provide the same quality of care to disabled patients that they give to nondisabled ones. Further, only 56.5% of these respondents strongly agreed that they welcomed patients with disabilities to come to their medical practices. Ironically, perhaps, 18.1% of the sample strongly agreed that our healthcare system often treats disabled patients unfairly. Iezzoni and colleagues argue that the presence of such biased views among medical practitioners could contribute to the persistent healthcare disparities that routinely affect people with disabilities, who comprise about one quarter of the country's population (CDC, 2022). Other investigators report similar levels of discomfort among healthcare workers about working with disabled patients (e.g., Peacock, 2019), including focusing only on the disability while ignoring related or accompanying health problems (Andrews, 2020).

Such biased attitudes toward people with disabilities are another form of disability stigma (recall Chapter 1). The insidious problem, of course, is that many of the very healthcare providers who should not have antipathy toward their disabled clients do harbor negative sentiments. In any case, the compounding problem is that such attitudes are also linked with low-quality healthcare outcomes for people with disabilities (Dovidio & Fiske, 2012; McColl et al., 2008). Some studies of spinal cord injury, for example, demonstrated that medical staff often view their patients as being more distressed and pessimistic where prognoses are concerned than the patients themselves are (Bodenhamer et al., 1983; Dijkers, 1997; Dijkers & Cushman, 1990; Ernst, 1987). Other research examined the responses of clients who had surgical "losses" (i.e., removal of some body part via amputation, colostomy, hysterectomy, or mastectomy) or the diagnosis of some terminal cancer along with the observations of their medical caregivers (i.e., physicians, nurses, nursing assistants, nursing students; Mason & Muhlenkamp, 1976). The latter consistently exaggerated the degree to which their clients were reporting negative affect (e.g., anxiety, hostility, depression) compared to the patients' own self-reports. Discrepancies between these emotional points of view were not a result of patient denial regarding the surgical losses, implying that medical staff were assuming (rather than verifying) the presence of poorer adjustment.

Wright (1987) believed that rehabilitation and medical professionals who work with disabled clients should acknowledge that such negative feelings toward clients can and do exist. As a result, professionals should routinely assess the quality of their interactions with clients to ensure that no biases are present and that they are behaving in a sensitive manner. Such careful and concerned *self-monitoring* is an essential way for professionals to maintain their clients' dignity. Doubtless, rehabilitation teams should also routinely check themselves to ensure that they are treating all clients with the same degree of attention and care.

Still, despite such professional scrutiny, negative thoughts, feelings, and behaviors may color judgment in particular ways.

HIERARCHICAL ATTITUDES AND DISABILITY

Nondisabled people—including professionals—may not realize they hold negative attitudes toward disability and disabled persons (such attitudes are referred to as *implicit*; Pruett & Chan, 2006; Robey et al., 2006). Attitudes can vary where such negativity is concerned. In fact, some forms of disabilities are viewed as being more acceptable than others. Physical disabilities are generally seen in more favorable terms than are mental disabilities, which are in turn viewed more positively than are intellectual disabilities; the lowest favorability ratings are associated with psychiatric disabilities (e.g., Chan et al., 2002, 2009; Tsang et al., 2004). This is especially true if those with psychiatric disabilities are seen as somehow being responsible for their conditions (Corrigan & Watson, 2002; Corrigan et al., 2000).

People with disabilities themselves are not immune to such negative feelings about disabilities (i.e., a form of internalized stigma). Deal (2003) found that some disabled people do not necessarily want to associate with other people with disabilities (neither like themselves nor with very different impairments). However, Deal also observed that disabled individuals who intentionally spent time with other people with disabilities held the most favorable attitudes toward disability (perhaps due to an appreciation for disability identity or connection with the disability community). Still, even among disabled people, internalized stereotypes and prejudices can influence feelings about the self and other disabled people (see Di Giulio, 2003).

The aforementioned hierarchical attitudes toward various types of disabilities are also found among disabled persons. Thus, physically disabled individuals or those with sensory disabilities see themselves as less stigmatized than those with intellectual, mental, or psychiatric disabilities (Deal, 2003; Chen et al., 2002). Andrews (2020) also suggested that some disabled persons avoid association, romance, or sexual partnership with other disabled persons, either within their disability group or with those with other types of disability.

Yet dignity is often found where people have a common cause or some shared experience. One representative example will be considered as a dignity source.

Dignity as Found in One Disability Community

The acclaimed film *Crip Camp* (Newman & LaBrecht, 2020) was mentioned in passing early on in Chapter 3. The film links an important avenue of the disability rights movement in the United States to Camp Jened, a summer camp in the Catskill Mountains of New York that offered a welcoming place for teenagers and young adults with various disabilities (including polio and cerebral palsy) from 1951 until 1977. For many of these campers, it was their first opportunity to meet and find common ground with other disabled youth in a judgment-free environment. The film relates the freedom they felt to be and to love themselves while also developing pride in their disabled status. One of the primary messages of *Crip Camp* is that many attendees found and felt their shared humanity and dignity there for the first time. Yet the film is not at all voyeuristic; rather, it introduces us to the everyday lives of many disabled teens, whose lived experience shows how their civil rights had been denied, their awakening to this fact, and the lifelong connections they quickly form that promote acceptance as well as ongoing activism.

Many campers, including the later-celebrated disability rights activist Judy Heumann (1947–2023), developed a drive to advocate for the rights of disabled people due to their summer camp experiences. The political pressure exerted by many former campers helped with the passage of the Americans with Disabilities Act (1990). *Crip Camp* illustrates the importance of creating a place and opportunity for people with disabilities to meet, organize, and campaign for their civil rights (recall the importance tied to the person-environment relation discussed in Chapter 3). As the film shows, being heard and taken seriously—that is, with respect and dignity—is a challenge but a welcome one. If nothing else, this positive documentary illustrates the important place and function that ad hoc disability communities (like Camp Jened) represent where establishing positive connections and relationships among disabled persons are concerned.

Camp Jened is but one setting that provided community and fomented activism. There are a variety of activist groups (e.g., Not Dead Yet) and other organizations that attract disabled people and channel their energies in constructive ways. The point is that fellowship and community can be important sources of dignity.

But these groups are specifically meant to attract disabled persons but not nondisabled ones. What can nondisabled people do in their daily lives to promote dignity for their disabled peers? How can they be effective allies who see the digntity of disabled persons in daily life as an important concern?

Providing Dignity in Daily Life: Recommendations for Interacting with Disabled Individuals

We know that many nondisabled people have had little to no experience with people with disabilities, which is one of the reasons that the foundational principles are so

TABLE 8.2

General Recommendations for First Encounters with Disabled Individuals
Curiosity is normal, but avoid asking about a disability unless the insider brings it up in conversation.
Don't talk about the disability unless the disabled person wants to do so.
Don't ask questions about a person's disability immediately—get to know them as a person first.
Consider the mood of the disabled individual.
Don't dwell on the disability; focus instead on the person.
Similarly, don't try to steer the person away from the subject of disability if they have a need to discuss it with you.
Avoid being solicitous; offer help only when asked or if the situation truly requires it.
Trying to "move things along" by expediting or assisting without being asked is usually not helpful and is often rude or even infantilizing.
Address the disabled person directly; don't ask an attendant or family member about the person's needs.
Be polite and exercise common courtesy; treat disabled people as you prefer to be treated.

Source: Adapted from Wright (1983 p. 306)

important. Very often, nondisabled people are uncertain how to behave, and often their anxiety or worry about doing the right thing backfires during social interactions, which can quickly become stilted and awkward. Such instances reinforce the stereotypes and ambivalent feelings harbored by both parties. Wright (1983) recognized this as a consequential social problem and, citing the work of White et al. (1948), offered some guidelines for first encounters with disabled individuals (see also Millington, 2012).

Naturally, the main goal is to treat disabled people with human dignity while also respecting their privacy and integrity (e.g., Dunn, 2015). Disabled people themselves should determine when and if any discussions concerning their conditions occur. Nondisabled individuals must follow the lead and wishes of their disabled peers, quelling their curiosity and desire to "know more." One unfortunate consequence of the expansion of social media is that the average person feels emboldened to ask what formerly would have been regarded as private or even impertinent questions in both online and in-person venues. The guidelines found in Table 8.2 are designed to temper or moderate social meetings while affording disabled people the dignity they deserve.

Certainly, rehabilitation and medical professionals can rely on these guidelines, as well, but they may also want to consult Olkin (1999) and Andrews' (2020) discussions of the cultural incompetencies that are often aimed at people with disabilities. Even professionals may not realize when their comments, demeanor, or behavior may send subtle or not so subtle messages of negativity or even microaggressions toward the disabled people they are trying to help or counsel.

Postscript on Human Dignity and Disability

I revisited this chapter after the August 2024 Democratic National Convention, because when Governor Tim Walz of Minnesota accepted the post as Kamala Harris's vice-presidential running mate during the convention, his 17-year-old, neurodiverse son, Gus Walz, was seen sobbing, clapping his hands, and happily exclaiming "That's my dad!" as his father delivered his address. Gus Walz was long ago diagnosed with a nonverbal learning disorder, ADHD (adult attention-deficit/hyperactivity disorder), as well as an anxiety disorder. His family has always viewed these qualities as Gus's "secret power" and embraced them. Regrettably, the conservative commentator Ann Coulter shared a tweet (on X) about Gus's behavior: "Talk about weird," along with a video of the boy. After being told Gus was disabled, Coulter deleted the tweet from her feed but did not apologize for her rude and insensitive comment.[1] Subsequently, other right-wing sources derided Gus's love of and enthusiasm for his father. Whether they did or did not know that he is neurodiverse does not matter.

We must always remember that disabled people—whether children or adults—are not things, just as ableism is sometimes subtle and other times obvious. In any case, disabled people's right to human dignity and to be treated with kindness and decency is and must be inviolate.

Precis and Prospects

Foundational principle 6 deals with the importance of recognizing and affirming the human dignity of people with disabilities. Human dignity was defined in general and with specific regard to disability contexts, the foundational principles, and the earlier value-laden beliefs and principles. The importance of focusing on the person, that is, the client's own experiences and worldviews, was emphasized. Such perspectives inform and guide the professional obligations and clinical work of both rehabilitation

1. This regrettable event echoes a November 26, 2015, event when then–presidential candidate Donald Trump publicly mocked a *New York Times* reporter, Serge Kovaleski.

and medical practitioners. Attitudinal challenges tied to professionals and disabled persons themselves, including the reality of negative attitudes toward disability and disabled people, were considered in detail. Dignity to be found in disabled groups and communities was discussed as a source of solace and activism, and then lay and professional approaches to effective communication with disabled people and clients were noted. In Chapter 9, the focus will be on advocacy efforts designed to help disabled people flourish. The seventh foundational principle promotes the view that advocacy is the responsibility of disabled individuals and their allies.

THOUGHT QUESTIONS

1. What is *human dignity*? Why is this an important aspect of understanding disability and the experience of being disabled?
2. Why is human dignity a fundamental right for all?
3. Why are myths and stereotypes of disability so prevalent and problematic?
4. Why is the word *person* an important consideration when discussing disability? How did this work influence the evolution of therapeutic work with clients, including disabled ones?
5. Why are professional obligations so important to work done with and for people with disabilities?
6. What are some subtle violations of dignity perpetrated by medical and other health professionals? Why are these violations of great concern? If medical professionals harbor negative attitudes toward disability, can anything be done to counter these beliefs?
7. Do hierarchical attitudes influence professionals as well as disabled people? How and why?
8. Why do opportunities for disabled people to connect with one another matter so much? Why is Camp Jened (where the documentary *Crip Camp* originated) an important example?
9. What are some practical and constructive ways to interact with people with disabilities that maintain their human dignity?

9 Principle 7

ADVOCACY: NOW AND ALWAYS

Foundational Principle 7: Advocacy Efforts

Advocacy efforts aimed at promoting the health and well-being of disabled individuals are important. Such efforts should be made by disabled people themselves as well as their allies (e.g., family, friends, medical and rehabilitation professionals).

> Acknowledging that advocacy efforts should take its place among the other six Foundational Principles is not only reasonable but meaningful action to remind disabled people and rehabilitation psychologists—practitioners, researchers, and educators—that disability is a form of diversity and that disabled individuals continue to seek equity within and inclusion in all spheres of society.
>
> —Andrews et al. (2023, p. 109)

> Nothing about us without us!
>
> —A slogan for Disability Rights

> Our mission is to lead the community of psychologists who, through research, practice, education and advocacy, enhance the well-being of people living with disability or chronic health conditions.
>
> —Mission Statement of APA Division 22 (Rehabilitation Psychology)

On the Foundational Principles of Rehabilitation Psychology. Dana S. Dunn, Oxford University Press.
 DOI: 10.1093/9780197785188.003.0009

This seventh foundational principle is the newest one. Advocacy efforts involve organizing support for a given cause or to advance some social policy. They can also entail gathering the backing of others to help you express your views or wishes tied to life experiences, opportunities, and even direction or destiny. Where disability is concerned, advocacy emerged from a client-based and professional consensus that disabled individuals cannot be expected to take on the structural and systemic challenges posed by the socio-political environment and ableist attitudes by themselves. Advocacy efforts should be based on collective action taken by disabled individuals and disability organizations and communities, as well as by lay and professional allies. When effective, advocacy can enable everyone to experience the common good (e.g., West, 2023).

Given the pressing need for advancing the interests of people with disabilities, adding advocacy as the most recent Foundational Principle is a reasonable course of action. Wright (1983) recommended that any guiding principles for the work done in rehabilitation psychology must be open to periodic review as well as occasional expansion. Given the important role advocacy plays in the collective lives of disabled persons, adding a seventh principle dedicated to it seems like an appropriate and timely expansion (Andrews et al., 2023). Advocacy represents not only a new foundational principle but a core competency of rehabilitation psychology. Specialty board certification, which is available through the American Board of Rehabilitation Psychology, considers advocacy to be a functional competency, one that requires candidates to display advocacy skills at both the individual patient level and as tied to disability issues more generally (American Board of Professional Psychology/American Board of Rehabilitation Psychology, 2022; Cox et al., 2013). Despite the importance of advocacy efforts and opportunities, however, rehabilitation professionals usually do not receive formal training or guidance in these matters (Andrews et al., 2023).

This chapter briefly reviews the history of advocacy in psychology, followed by consideration of relevant efforts involving disability, disabled persons, and rehabilitation psychology. The nature of disability research as a form of advocacy is then considered, highlighting the challenges in doing authentic work that actively involves insiders as consultants and researchers as well as the slow adoption of a new research paradigm. One response to the latter concern is the use of participatory action research (PAR), or more simply, action research, which champions culturally competent approaches to disability. Although rehabilitation psychology has a history of helping disabled people become independent and self-sufficient, what the disability community needs to do is leverage its interdependence. Crucial examples of disability advocacy during the COVID-19 pandemic are then reviewed, followed by disability justice matters as a forum for advocacy efforts. The chapter closes by focusing on priorities for disability advocacy and disability justice, as well as identifying levels of advocacy and topics therein.

Advocacy in Psychology: A Brief History

Many years ago, the then-president of the American Psychological Association, experimental psychologist George A. Miller (1969), suggested that members of the field should work hard to "give psychology away." By that, he meant that the discipline had a choice to make: It could develop and hold onto specialized scientific knowledge, or it could aim to share beneficial scientific insights with the public to improve the quality of daily life. Miller argued in favor of the latter position, and to a considerable degree, his vision is being achieved. Psychology courses are popular at the undergraduate level (introductory psychology is the second most popular course after the first-year writing course; Gurung & Neufeld, 2022), and there is evidence of continued growth and interest in the psychological literacy of the public (Banyard & Hulme, 2015). Psychology also remains one of the most popular undergraduate majors. Findings from psychological science journals are routinely turned into popularized versions that make their way into various social media where they are generally well received by consumers. Finally, whether they are practitioners, researchers, or educators (or some combination thereof), psychologists are recognized as helpful resources for both private and public life.

Although Miller did not necessarily have rehabilitation psychology or the needs of people with disabilities spelled out in his provocative article (see the exchange between Miller [1970] and Myers [1970]), he might as well have done so, because leveraging scientific knowledge in ways that improve people's lives is at the heart of what is done in this subfield of psychology. In a special issue of the *American Psychologist* dedicated to public psychology, Neville et al. (2021) highlighted a speech given at the 1967 APA convention by Dr. Martin Luther King, Jr. In his remarks, Dr. King observed that the discipline of psychology usually focuses on how individuals adjust to situations. However, during his speech, King claimed that he would be proud to be labeled maladjusted where certain things, such as racial segregation, discrimination, and religious bigotry, were concerned. Andrews et al. (2023) suggested Dr. King would likely also add ableism to his maladjustment list were he alive today. Indeed, psychology has generally continued to focus on individual adjustment while overlooking the influence of the contexts and social environments where it occurs (cf., Chapter 3; Dunn, 2019c; Lewin, 1935; Wright, 1983). At the same time, calls for advancing social justice interests in psychology have been issued by feminists, people of color, disabled psychologists, and LGBTQI+ colleagues—despite the fact that these very groups were long marginalized within the discipline.

The COVID-19 pandemic also revealed sociopolitical agendas and unfair health disparities tied to social justice issues (e.g., Andrews et al., 2021; Bhattarai et al., 2020; Lund, 2021; Lund & Ayers, 2020; Lund et al., 2020), a topic to be discussed later in this chapter. Advocacy, then, is a means for psychologists to tackle social justice issues, which have a long history in the field of rehabilitation psychology.

ADVOCACY IN REHABILITATION PSYCHOLOGY

> Research that produces nothing but books will not suffice.
>
> —Kurt A. Lewin (1997, p. 144)

As this quote from Lewin suggests, though important, psychological research is of little use beyond providing intellectual interest unless it is applied to create useful changes and meaningful improvements in the world. That perspective is at the heart of rehabilitation psychology. Rehabilitation psychology became a profession that developed during and grew after World War II (Larson & Sachs, 2000), and its current mission statement (shown at the opening of this chapter) is explicit about the importance of advocacy efforts. Such efforts have always been a part of the rehabilitative process and this subfield of psychology. US veterans returning home required many medical, social, and educational services, which allowed psychologists to provide academic, vocational, guidance, and counseling assistance. These efforts helped former soldiers to re-enter and begin the process of adjusting to civilian life, in many cases with acquired disabilities. Various public policy initiatives were enacted that were designed to help people with disabilities and the professionals now working in fields that served their requirements (Rusalem, 1976). Later, the Vocational Rehabilitation Act of 1954 helped to sponsor necessary academic training of psychologists to meet the vocational rehabilitation needs of disabled people. Advocacy in the form of identifying and satisfying the needs of people with disabilities has always been a mainstay effort in Division 22.

Practice was clearly an early concern for rehabilitation psychology, but what about theory? As noted earlier in this book, social psychological theories, especially those developed by Kurt Lewin and his students, including Beatrice Wright and Tamara Dembo, as well as the work of Roger Barker, created early guidelines for working with disabled persons as well as a foundation for rehabilitation psychology. At the same time, the work of clinical, counseling, and humanistic psychologists (recall Chapter 8), including Carl Rogers, Abraham Maslow, and Kenneth Spence, also helped the fledgling discipline (Dunn & Elliott, 2005; see also, Dunn & Elliott, 2008). And, as we have learned in this book, the Foundational Principles embody theory, empirical, and practice perspectives.

But what about research and how it was—and is now—conceived and conducted?

THE NATURE OF DISABILITY RESEARCH

On its face, disability-related research may not seem to be linked to advocacy. However, one persistent fact suggests that it should be: Across time, research on disability has been conducted primarily by nondisabled academics rather than disabled researchers (Kitchin, 2000). This fact remains true today, though it seems that more disabled researchers are now active in the field. Ehde et al. (2013) noted this disconnection between research on disability issues and the involvement of members of the disability community. In other words, one important aspect of advocacy entails involving disabled people in research efforts—not only as participants or consumers of such research, but as creators, investigators, and consultants. One of the main messages of the foundational principles is that the perspectives and knowledge of disabled people should be an important part of practice and treatment. Logically, it seems that the tools used in practice and treatment are likely based on research—so insider perspectives should not only inform but often actively guide or direct such research.

Perhaps the history and evolution of rehabilitation research should not be a surprise at this juncture. As Andrews (2020) notes, most research on disability issues relied on the medical model, so that disabled participants (then known as "subjects," a term that has fallen out of favor due to its objectifying quality) were the focus of study (Stodden et al., 2003). Such research was based in clinic settings or hospitals where the goals were diagnosis, treatment, and where possible, prevention of disability (McDonald & Raymaker, 2013; Scotch, 2002).

Over 35 years ago, in the *Journal of Social Issues*, Fine and Asch (1988) argued that most disability research still primarily addressed medical aspects of disability, an impairment-oriented approach that highlighted presumed needs and interventions tied to help and social support. The "stigma" of disability was the driver of theory and research, and the critique identified a subtext of meaning where disabled people were portrayed as victims of circumstance. More to the point, their disabilities were seen as central to their lived experience—all other aspects of their identities or assets were downplayed or even ignored (for example, recall Chapters 1 and 6). Fine and Asch called for greater social interaction and integration for disabled people, recognition of the discrimination they face(d), and increased activism—which naturally included an advocacy component.

As Andrews (2020) observed, it took almost 20 years for interest in a new paradigm for disability research to emerge (Gill et al., 2003; Olkin & Pledger, 2003; Tate & Pledger, 2003), one that would replace the medical model. The main change was to portray disability as a social construct while relying on the social model of disability to advance research that had social and political ramifications. And instead of always focusing on the individual experience of disability, that is, as a personal phenomenon, Olkin and Pledger (2003) promoted examining the societal, familial, and political sides of the disability experience. Specific research challenges they identified included these four points:

1. *Much current research continues a "we-they" divide.* Most researchers are outsiders, and most research participants are insiders. This reality does not negate the contributions of nondisabled colleagues; rather, it calls attention to the need for more balanced membership on research teams.
2. *Disability-related research is one of the few topics examining minority experiences that has few minorities (insiders) leading research efforts.* For example, those who examine ethnicity, race, ageism, women's issues, and sexual orientation typically represent the groups they study. The underrepresentation of people with disabilities points to legitimate structural and conceptual questions regarding the validity of the work.
3. *Despite the emphasis on the person-environment relation (foundational principle 1), many existing research efforts do not embrace disability as a problem tied to civil rights or economic, social, and legal concerns.* Too often, disability is portrayed as a problem of the individual rather than being addressed at the group level of analysis; put another way, the figure and not the ground remains the primary focus of research (recall Chapter 3).
4. *The bulk of disability and rehabilitation research neglects disability history and culture by concentrating on treatment (usually acute) issues, as well as adjustment and adaptation.* Remnants of the medical model and the tendency to pathologize linger despite the push to view disability from societal, chronic, and life span perspectives or those linked to positive psychology (see Chapter 6).

For a more detailed comparison of the older (medical model) and newer (social or minority model) paradigms, please see Table 2 in Olkin and Pledger (2003, p. 301).

Still, to some extent, whether intentional or not, psychological research on disability began to borrow ideas from disability studies, a field that soundly rejects the idea that any or all disabilities should be "cured." As Siebers (2011) put it,

> Disability studies does not treat disease or disability, hoping to cure or avoid them; it studies the social meanings, symbols, and stigmas attached to disability identity and asks how they relate to enforced systems of exclusion and oppression, attacking the widespread belief that having an able body and mind determines whether one is a quality human being. (pp. 3–4)

Thus, the advocacy message inherent in the newer paradigm and disability studies calls for reliance on approaches that promote more active involvement of insiders and the disability community in order create culturally competent research. As Andrews (2020) observed, "Disabled people deserve to see others like themselves in these roles and have the chance to fill them" (p. 167).

Advancing Culturally Competent Research Efforts

Andrews (2020) identified PAR as an appropriate framework for conducting culturally competent research efforts dealing with disability issues. Even though it has not been a popular method in rehabilitation psychology research, its history and scope are linked to the first generation of rehabilitation theorists (see Ehde et al., 2013; Nelson et al., 1998). Often used in fields like public health, human geography, and creative arts practice, as well as in educational research, PAR is based on the action research efforts of Kurt Lewin and his early students (Torre et al., 2012). PAR uses both qualitative and quantitative methods. Following Lewin, PAR presumes that the best way to truly understand social systems is to implement changes within them (Nelson et al., 1998). Our discussion of Dembo's insider-outsider distinction (see Chapter 4) highlights the acquired perspectives tied to the lived experience of disability (or the lack thereof), a key point of participatory efforts.

Still, there is no one set definition of action research or PAR. Lewin is the titular "father" of PAR and other forms of action research due to his practical lab and field experiments designed and conducted to deal with practical challenges before and during World War II (Maruyama & Van Boekel, 2014). Lewin believed that experts in theory (researchers) could work with and learn from experts in practice (practitioners and others who know a subject intimately, including through lived experience; see, for example, Lewin, 1946). Such theory and practice partnerships were established to go through several cycles of planning (i.e., hypothesis generation),

TABLE 9.1

Core Aspects of PAR for Disability
Consumer involvement: Disabled stakeholders shape all phases of the research process.
Cooperation: Disabled and nondisabled people involved in a research project share in decision-making and mutually own the project and its direction.
Empowerment: PAR respects disabled consumers, knowing they will use their valuable knowledge and experience to improve the disability community.
Facilitation of change: PAR for disability advances sociopolitical transformation, especially where public policy and health issues are concerned, identifying who might benefit, be harmed, or be put at risk.

Source: Adapted from Andrews (2020, p. 168)

action (i.e., intervention, such as attitude change), fact finding (i.e., data collection), and then a report on the process to review the problem and the results (e.g., Aguinis, 1993). Often, following such a review, the stages are refined, and the cycle is repeated to learn more about the topic being studied.

A detailed discussion of how to do PAR is beyond the scope of our current discussion (for a more detailed review, see Andrews, 2020; Torre et al., 2012). PAR and other forms of action research can be done and defined in a variety of ways (e.g., Blair & Minkler, 2009; Cassell & Johnson, 2006; Conder et al., 2011; Maciver et al., 2013; Torre et al., 2012), but they all share the four core tenets found in Table 9.1: consumer involvement, cooperation, empowerment, and facilitating change. PAR efforts involve disabled colleagues (i.e., consumers or clients) in all stages of the project—from conception to writing and publication. As members or leaders of the research team, insiders have a serious stake in the PAR project's success as well as the right to approve or veto what is done during the project. As active partners in PAR, insiders are recognized as possessing valuable experiences and information that can improve the lives of disabled people near and far. Finally, PAR is about understanding and causing change, particularly transformations that alter the sociopolitical and economic tenor of disabled people's lived experience.

Much well-intentioned research on disability issues and rehabilitation psychology focused on advancing the independence and self-sufficiency of disabled persons (Andrews, 2020). Although these appear to be laudable goals, as values, they are not culturally competent or necessarily representative of the point of view of the disability community, which often celebrates the interdependence of its members. As we learned in Chapter 2, as the largest minority group in the United States (and likely elsewhere, too), disabled people must be understood in terms of their intersectionality, which means varieties of diversity (e.g., racial, ethnic, religious, cultural, linguistic, LGBTQ+) as well as collectivist rather than individualistic (i.e., Western, White American, or otherwise WEIRD[1]) views. To advance more culturally appropriate and sensitive research that involved diverse peoples, Berghs et al. (2016) created the IDEAS decision aid tool (which considers issues of inclusion, dignity, equity, accessibility, and intersectionality) for advancing cultural competence in disability research. Andrews (2020) presented the IDEAS approach as a research checklist, an adaptation of which appears in Table 9.2. When developing any research project involving disabled people (ideally as researchers, consultants, and participants), a review of the framework, questions, and issues presented in Table 9.2 should guide the discussion to ensure that obvious or obscured sociopolitical issues are recognized so that interpretative influence is moderated appropriately.

In some sense, advocacy efforts on behalf of disabled persons were tested during the COVID-19 pandemic, which began in earnest in the spring of 2020. Research efforts in rehabilitation psychology highlighted the concerns and challenges that arose as the United States and other countries around the world entered a lockdown period.

An Exemplar: Disability Advocacy During the COVID-19 Pandemic

As the pandemic spread, the health threats posed by the novel coronavirus were keenly felt by members of the disability community (e.g., Ne'eman, 2020). Many disabled people were vulnerable to exposure and the resulting health consequences tied to COVID-19. For example, some disabilities, but not all, put people at higher risk for infection and complications. Disabled people living in institutional settings, group and nursing homes, and assisted living facilities were at high risk due to the confining nature of the settings (i.e., rapid spread of the virus). Similarly, caregivers—family, friends, medical professionals and staff—were or could be potential carriers of the virus. Disabled people living independently had great difficulty protecting and sometimes caring for themselves through the necessary self-isolation. Such isolation was linked with depression and anxiety among disabled adults (Wang et al., 2022). In addition, when disabled persons were also members of marginalized racial and ethnic groups, their anxieties and stress regarding the pandemic were further heightened (Lund, 2021; Lund et al., 2020).

Andrews et al. (2021) described how shortages of medical equipment led to the establishment of triage guidelines indicating how any available equipment, including

1. This acronym, coined by Heinrich et al. (2010), refers to Western, educated, industrialized, rich, and democratically oriented people.

TABLE 9.2

Questions for Ensuring Cultural Competence in Research on Disability

Inclusion

Will the research engage in coproduction or involve disabled stakeholders when developing research questions and designs?

What are the implications of participation?

Dignity

Does the research reflect the diversity of disability?

How does it connect to the lived experiences of disabled people?

Does the research design take disability sensitivity into account?

What are the ethical considerations?

Are the theoretical and empirical implications of using particular types of measures explicit?

Equity:

How does the research improve the health and well-being of people with a range of different impairments, conditions, and/or mental health issues?

Does the research link to social entitlements for well-being and/or enabling social environments?

What disability model(s) inform the research?

How well does the research reflect the actual experience of disability? If not, is this made clear?

Accessibility

Is the intervention and study designed with accessibility in mind?

How can accessibility be ensured?

Are any disabled participants needlessly excluded?

How well does the research engage people who use nonverbal communication, have cognitive impairments, and/or learning disabilities, for example?

Intersectionality

Does existing evidence indicate a gap in the literature on health inequalities?

How well does the research link to intersectionality and comorbidities?

How does it connect to age, gender, socioeconomic status, sexuality, disability, ethnicity, geography, or other pertinent factors?

Analytical framework

How well does the research characterize disability experiences that can connect to the theory/causal framework driving the intervention?

TABLE 9.2 *Continued*

Will disability-oriented recommendations emerge from the research or intervention?

Does the work promote examples of disabled people flourishing rather than having unfavorable outcomes?

Are explanations tied to disabling social and political environments considered?

Source: Adapted from Andrews (2020, pp. 178–179)

mechanical ventilators and intensive care unit beds, would be allocated. Triage guidelines—the assignment of degrees of urgency to wounds or illnesses, as well as selecting who is helped and who is not—means that some patients are prioritized over others, who receive no aid. Disabled people worried that they could be passed over, seen as a lower priority than nondisabled people (i.e., an incidence of medical ableism; see also Lund & Ayers, 2020). Medical rationing occurs when resources are limited, and medical resources are generally always finite (Brody, 2012). In addition, even when there are several potentially beneficial treatments at hand, there is no certainty that a given treatment will actually help a particular patient. Health care providers must always balance the costs and benefits of any chosen medical intervention to justify the expense of using it. Yet serious worries exist, as some rationing appeared to unfairly discriminate against disabled people as well as those with chronic health conditions. The transplantation of organs, for example, is still denied based on the presence of disability alone (Chen et al., 2020; for other examples, see Andrews et al., 2021).

The Disability Rights Movement has a long history of disagreement with the field of bioethics. Some bioethicists (e.g., Peter Singer, a philosopher at Princeton University; see McBryde Johnson, 2003, 2005) argue that disabled newborns should not be provided with lifesaving treatment and that euthanizing them is both permissible and merciful. This sort of logic explains triage protocols that might reject disabled people from treatment (e.g., "Why waste equipment or bedspace on someone who is likely to die?"). Yet as we have seen, ample research from rehabilitation psychology and disability studies demonstrates that the presence of disability *does not* predict a poor quality of life or preclude a healthy one (see also Bishop et al., 2024).

How do advocacy efforts fit into this clearly challenging arena? To begin, reducing implicit biases where medical resources are concerned is essential, which means that no frontline medical providers should be making such ethically fraught decisions. Medical professionals at all levels need to be made aware of ableism and its consequences for fairness in medical triage and resource allocations. Such education needs to ensure understanding beyond disability as a medical status but also as a social, political, and lived experience, one that is subject to intentional and unintentional ableism. For example, disabled persons routinely encountered barriers to obtaining needed mental health services during the COVID-19 pandemic (Manning et al., 2023). Differentiating among equality (everyone is treated equally), equity (individual needs are met), and justice (removal of systematic barriers and illumination of the cause of initial inequities) is necessary. Addressing the intersectionality associated with disability is also important, as it connects to gender, age, income, race, and LGBTQ issues, among others (recall Chapter 2).

Who decides? Committees composed of interdisciplinary experts, including disabled representatives, should be the ones developing future rationing policies and triage guidelines. As Andrews et al. (2021) pointed out, research conducted by the Centers for Disease Control (CDC) on COVID-19 should collect demographic data so relevant analyses can determine how, whether, and when disability plays a role in health outcomes. At the same time, disabled people need both representation and participation in ethical decisions regarding how medical resources are used.

Finally, we often forget that health is socially determined. In the United States, for example, only 10 to 15% of preventable mortality is linked with medical care (see Andrews et al., 2021). The way people live—their lifestyles, choices, and behaviors matter a great deal to their well-being. Various social factors, including education, income, and employment, affect beneficial health outcomes (or the lack thereof; see McGinnis & Foege, 1993). Five key domains are influential where health and well-being are concerned: economic stability, education, health and health care, neighborhood and built environment, and social and community context (see Andrews et al., 2021). As we have observed, in each of these contexts, disabled persons are more likely to experience disadvantages than are their nondisabled peers.

Developing lines of disability advocacy and highlighting social justice issues before there is another public health crisis like the COVID-19 pandemic would seem to be prudent.

Priorities for Disability Advocacy and Disability Justice

What matters where priorities for disability advocacy are concerned, now and in the future? There is not much that is either new or news here. Most people with disabilities live in impoverished circumstances. Although disability is recognized as a form of diverse human experience, widespread ableism (prejudice and discrimination, whether active or passive) still violates the inherent dignity and worth of disabled people. Disabled persons are more likely to experience structural barriers (social, attitudinal, physical, economic) than nondisabled people. Moreover, although a desire to advance human rights exists, there are many disabled people who need but do not receive intensive support (Andrews et al., 2023). Within the disability community, particular subgroups are especially prone to experiencing discrimination, including people of color, indigenous persons, disabled children, and women and girls who have disabilities.

Clearly, and as Andrews et al. (2023) reminded rehabilitation psychologists, disabled persons constitute a heterogeneous population (recall Chapter 2), a fact that makes choosing and articulating public policy priorities for advocacy a real challenge. Yet a group of artist performers who are disability advocates—known as Sins Invalid—crafted a living and dynamic list of 10 principles for disability justice (Berne et al., 2018). Shown in Table 9.3, these principles lay out advocacy points that were generated by and for the disability community. They resist historic calls for charity and a focus on medical or diagnostic issues while recognizing the importance of disability identity, intersectionality, and other more pressing sociopolitical concerns. Disabled people and their allies, including rehabilitation and medical professionals, should rely on these principles when advocating for issues and causes tied to disability rights, social justice issues, and public policy initiatives.

LEVELS OF ADVOCACY

Miles and Fassinger (2021) argued that the best advocacy for the field of psychology can only occur by adopting a scientist-practitioner-advocate (SPA) training model. These authors identified four levels of advocacy: individual, institutional, discipline, and community. Miles and Fassinger noted, "The primary goals of the SPA model are reimagining of the roles of scientist, practitioner, and advocate as essential, interlocking aspects of a psychologist identity, and the development of a social justice orientation across these roles (p. 1242)." Without training, mentoring, and other forms of encouragement, however, it is unlikely that students or established professionals will use their skills to advance the public good.

Fortunately, to a certain degree, rehabilitation psychologists and colleagues in allied fields already have some training and a social justice orientation toward disability and people with disabilities. With further guidance and support, they are poised to be effective advocates for change, particularly if they adopt the view that partnering with disabled individuals and the larger disability community is the best way to achieve desired outcomes. Andrews et al. (2023) outline a variety of disability

TABLE 9.3

The 10 Principles of Disability Justice

1. *Intersectionality*, or the acknowledgement that the experience of disability is shaped by other identities,
2. *Leadership of the Most Impacted*, which are disabled people of color,
3. *Anti-Capitalism*, or a resistance to conforming to capitalist notions of White supremacy, gender normativity, and expectations of productivity at the expense of health,
4. *Cross-Movement Solidarity*, or engagement in non-disability advocacy for human rights,
5. *Recognizing Wholeness*, or valuing people for who they are with their inherent worth,
6. *Sustainability*, or understanding the need to rest and sustain efforts for long-term progress,
7. *Commitment to Cross-Disability Solidarity*, or honoring participation of all community members through universal access,
8. *Interdependence*, or the intentional preferences for working together in the face of Western glorification of independence,
9. *Collective Access*, or celebrating our strengths while exercising creativity in meeting access needs, and
10. *Collective Liberation*, or a collective commitment to leave no disabled body or mind behind.

Source: Andrews et al. (2023, Table 2; text by Sins Invalid)

advocacy opportunities at the individual, institutional, and discipline levels that can be linked to relevant policy matters and policymakers. Some examples suggesting how advocacy can be encouraged and performed at all three levels are listed in Table 9.4. Readers are encouraged to use these suggested opportunities to advocate for disabled people, just as they are urged to expand the entries within each category.

Precis and Prospects

This chapter provided an overview of the history of advocacy in psychology, followed by efforts tied to disability and rehabilitation psychology. The nature of disability research as a form of advocacy was then discussed, highlighting work that

TABLE 9.4

Disability Advocacy Opportunities at the Individual, Institutional, and Discipline Levels

Individual Level
Working with clients and families
Forming interdisciplinary teams
Working in inpatient and outpatient settings
Explaining and confronting ableism in practice and in professional settings
Teaching about disability, diverse disabilities, and disability as diversity
Pursuing administrative and leadership positions in healthcare settings
Serving as training directors and supervisors in rehabilitation psychology
Pursuing inclusive research and scientific inquiry
Institutional Level
Advancing organizational commitments to disability and disability diversity
Eliminating ableist bylaws and organizational inequities
Creating nondiscriminatory hiring practices and recruiting diverse applicants
Ensuring that human rights and social justice themes appear in curricula and courses
Emphasizing PAR methodologies in research and scholarship
Providing advocacy skills training for professionals and trainees
Discipline Level
Creating discipline-wide standards for education and training, human rights, and social justice advocacy
Helping disabled students and trainees become rehabilitation psychologists
Modeling inclusivity and accessibility
Diversifying the editors and editorial boards of specialty journals
Making interdependence become a value associated with rehabilitation psychology

Source: Adapted from Andrews et al. (2023)

actively involves insiders as consultants and researchers as well as a new research paradigm. Participatory action research (PAR) was identified as a culturally competent method for studying disability issues. The dire need for disability advocacy during the COVID-19 pandemic was then considered, as were disability justice matters as a forum for advocacy efforts. The chapter concluded by focusing on priorities for disability advocacy and disability justice, as well as identifying levels of advocacy for individuals, institutions, and the wider discipline. The next chapter—the final one in this book—discusses why the foundational principles are an important part of rehabilitation therapies and practice efforts and urges readers to use and cite the principles in their scholarship, teaching, practice, and advocacy efforts.

THOUGHT QUESTIONS

1. What is advocacy? Why are advocacy efforts important for disabled people and the wider disability community?
2. Why should advocacy efforts tied to disability become the seventh foundational principle?
3. How have practice, theory, and research efforts in rehabilitation psychology advanced advocacy efforts for disabled persons?
4. How has research on disability and disabled persons evolved across time? Why has the evolution been so slow? What are the four research challenges identified by Olkin and Pledger (2003)? Do these challenges remain concerns for research on disability and in rehabilitation psychology?
5. Why does participant action research (PAR) represent a culturally competent approach to research on disability?
6. Why was disability advocacy so needed during the COVID-19 pandemic?
7. What are some examples of opportunities targeting the individual, institutional, and disciplinary levels of disability advocacy?

10 The Primacy of the Foundational Principles

> A lodestar is something, or someone, that provides guidance or inspiration, particularly to a group of people. The term is an apt one for our "Foundational Principles," based on Beatrice Wright's (1983) and other leaders' classic works, which guide the empirical research, theory, and practice in rehabilitation psychology.
>
> —Dunn et al. (2016, p. 1)

> The Foundational Principles play an important role in the history of rehabilitation psychology, as they have guided theory development, scholarly inquiry, and informed practice. But their true value lies in the manner in which they inform our current and future work as rehabilitation psychologists and lead to improved QoL [quality of life] for people with disabilities.
>
> —Dunn et al. (2016, p. 5)

ONE OF THE main purposes of this book is to remind readers—practitioners, therapists, scholars, researchers, students, lay people—that rehabilitation psychology is dedicated to exploring the psychological, biological, environmental, social, and political factors that affect the well-being and lives of individuals with disabilities and other chronic health conditions. Rehabilitation psychology endorses and accepts the biopsychosocial model of health (e.g., Leventhal et al., 2006) as well as the WHO

On the Foundational Principles of Rehabilitation Psychology. Dana S. Dunn, Oxford University Press.
© Oxford University Press (2025). DOI: 10.1093/9780197785188.003.0010

International Classification of Functioning, Disability, and Heath (ICF) model (World Health Organization, 2001; recall Chapter 1; see also Dunn, 2015, 2019b). To these ends, the foundational principles hold pride of place—that is, they represent a primary focus for professionals and interested others who seek a framework for science and practice issues tied to rehabilitation psychology and disability.

As Dunn et al. (2016) observed, to some extent, the foundational principles have always been an implicit part of the field of rehabilitation psychology. The goal of this book and related works is to render them explicit, thereby highlighting the key theoretical and clinical traditions of this subfield. Their utility should not be limited to the rehabilitation sciences, as psychological science generally, health services research, health policy studies, and public health and nursing might also benefit from making their acquaintance.

The seven foundational principles (see Table 1.1 in Chapter 1) are a distillation of Wright's value-laden beliefs and principles (Wright, 1972, 1983, 1993; Shontz & Wright, 1980) as well as an extension of them. As noted earlier, the relative brevity of the principles grants them a heuristic quality—that is, they should be relatively easy to recall and, therefore, readily applicable to situations that involve people with disabilities or chronic health issues. At the same time, the principles are meant to be flexible, really a "living" set of guidelines that should be subject to (following the lead of Beatrice A. Wright) ongoing evaluation, revision, and even addition as needed. They are not necessarily designed to be permanent; rather, like the field of rehabilitation psychology and its companion areas of inquiry—the social psychology of disability and disability studies—the principles should evolve and change to reflect theoretical, empirical, and therapeutic advances, as well as social change.

We will now consider how the foundational principles can connect to key issues tied to disability and rehabilitation psychology.

Some Foundational Touchstones

In the chapters devoted to each of the seven foundational principles (i.e., Chapters 3 to 9), we already explored how each one can be leveraged for understanding a relevant experience or aspect of disability and the rehabilitative process. We should not repeat much of that available information here. Instead, it is wiser to elucidate links to other important matters—or what we might call foundational touchstones. The term "touchstone" refers to a quintessential or even fundamental part or feature of something—its basis, as it were. It can also be a test or a criterion for deciding the quality or authenticity of a thing. In this section, we review some touchstones that are or should prove to be important arenas wherein the principles operate or can be applied. We begin with education and training as a key touchstone.

EDUCATION AND TRAINING

An obvious goal for establishing greater awareness and reliance on the foundational principles is teaching them to students interested in rehabilitation psychology and disability. Stiers (2016), for example, suggested that Wright's (1983) 20 value-laden beliefs and principles (as precursors to the current principles) should inform the education and training of rehabilitation psychologists through both content and teaching methods (see also Stiers, 2019). Graduate students in rehabilitation psychology should recognize and accept the principles as an important aspect of their training as well to acquire attitudes and values that promote the work done in this subfield. Stiers grouped the principles into three categories for explication: individual psychological processes, social psychological processes, and values tied to social integration. The result is a proposed core curriculum, including exemplar assignments for teaching the foundational principles to reduce prejudiced attitudes toward people with disabilities. Andrews's (2020) suggestions for developing cultural competence regarding disability and diversity issues could readily support and augment the material identified by Stiers.

Similarly, Tackett and colleagues (2016) argued that the foundational principles, as well as Wright's (1983) value-laden beliefs and principles, could inform clinical supervision of students during training. Although the specialty training in rehabilitation psychology requires exposure to specific knowledge, skills, and attitudes related to disability and specialized supervision and mentorship, Tackett and colleagues observed that minimal guidance recommendations can be found in the extant literature. Clinical supervision situations can serve as teaching vignettes aimed at promoting discussion between mentors and their students. Tackett et al.'s recommendations can promote discussion regarding practice issues and the dissemination of the values fundamental to rehabilitation psychology.

Another goal linked to education and training should be to make undergraduate students interested in psychology aware of issues regarding disability, the experience of people with disabilities, and the purpose and scope of rehabilitation psychology. The American Psychological Association's (APA's) Introductory Psychology Initiative seeks to make this first course in psychology transformational for students who enroll in it (and in the United States, over a million do each academic year; see Gurung & Neufeld, 2022; see also Richmond et al., 2021). A key goal of evidence-based course design for the introductory course is to promote inclusion by highlighting diversity issues. The popularity of the course ensures that it often attracts a wide variety of students who "vary in race, gender, age, disability, socioeconomic background, political views, and interests and goals" (Hard et al., 2022, p. 44).[1] However, few, if any, courses in the undergraduate psychology curriculum teach students about disability and issues of chronic illness, let alone introduce topics tied to rehabilitation psychology and its theories and therapeutic goals.

Still, since disabled people represent the largest minority group in the United States (recall Chapter 2), it would seem reasonable that undergraduate psychology majors should learn that fact while also exploring disability as a form of diversity (e.g., Andrews, 2020; Dunn, 2009, 2016; Dunn, Fisher, & Beard, 2013; Dunn & Hammer, 2014). In other words, the course content of introductory psychology is one place for greater diversification to occur, though it might be constructive to identity other courses that frequently appear in the undergraduate curriculum (e.g., core courses [e.g., social psychology], capstone courses, seminars) for additional diversification. Doing so will not only broaden undergraduate students' knowledge of the wider discipline, but the course content can also serve to promote a sense of community among students (Hard et al., 2022).

TIES TO POSITIVE PSYCHOLOGY

In early 2000s, the subfield known as *positive psychology* emerged as a new area for theorizing and empirical inquiry. One of the main goals of positive psychology is to identify, explore, and apply human strengths to help people flourish both psychologically and physically (e.g., Aspinwall & Staudinger, 2003; Keyes & Haidt, 2003; Peterson & Seligman, 2004; Seligman & Czsikszentmihalyi, 2000). Positive psychology was developed as a reaction to well-established but largely pathology-focused research (e.g., anxiety, depression) regarding human experience found in much of mainstream psychology and psychiatry. Instead, this young subfield searches for and promotes qualities and factors that maintain health, well-being, and positive outlooks and behaviors among people and among different age groups.

Positive psychology developed rapidly; books, handbooks, and dedicated journals appeared, followed by graduate programs that granted degrees in positive psychology. Not surprisingly, rehabilitation psychologists took notice and began to integrate concepts and constructs from positive psychology into their research and practice efforts. Dunn and Dougherty (2005), for example, claimed that prospects for a positive psychology of rehabilitation were quite good, because the scope of rehabilitation

1. Introductory Psychology is the most frequently taken course after first-year writing (or another introductory English course) within undergraduate general education curricula.

psychology has always included a focus on the health and well-being of clients. These authors reviewed rehabilitation psychology's positive core strengths, articulated positive psychology's levels of analysis and their implications for rehabilitation psychology, discussed subjective experiences following disability to illustrate positive rehabilitation psychology, examined some of the integrative positive models for research and practice, and outlined some positive resources for rehabilitation psychologists. As already discussed in Chapter 6, Dunn and Brody (2008) subsequently considered how positive psychology's perspectives could inform and lead to a "good life" following acquired physical disability.

Various topics tied to positive psychology, such as resilient reactions to disability or posttraumatic growth following disabling experiences, have been explored by rehabilitation psychologists, as well as researchers interested in disability (see, for example, Andrews et al., in press; Dunn, 2018, 2019a; Wehmeyer, 2013; Wehmeyer & Dunn, 2022b). Opportunities for research efforts tied to disability and human flourishing, well-being, quality of life, and related constructs abound. The ease with which positive psychology interests have aligned so well with rehabilitation and disability researchers is likely due to the tradition of support for disabled people and their families that is so well established in rehabilitation psychology (recall the Division 22 Mission Statement, which can be found in Chapter 9 on page 130). Certainly, use of the foundational principles and their positive perspectives will continue to advance a positive psychology for disability and rehabilitation.

THE ONGOING IMPORTANCE OF APPRAISAL PROCESSES

Attributional processes are at the heart of the social psychology of disability, as they inform how disabled and nondisabled people mutually assess one another in social interactions (Dunn, 2015). In addition, self-appraisal in the form of possessing, developing, articulating, and sharing one's disability identity is also an important example of appraisal (e.g., Dunn & Burcaw, 2013; Forber-Pratt et al., in press). Such subjective assessments, whether oriented toward the self or others, have important consequences for health and well-being.

Rehabilitation researchers and practitioners should not forget that the perception and recognition of stress, including that linked to disability, is also subjective. The foundational principles, notably principles 2 (the insider-outsider distinction) and 5 (self-perception of bodily states), embody and apply such subjective analyses. At the same time, we should not forget that appraisal processes highlight the importance of individual differences. What is stressful or threatening to one person may be acceptably routine for another, an important message found in the stress and coping theories of Richard Lazarus and Susan Folkman (1984; see also Folkman, 2010).

Lazarus and Folkman (1984) distinguished between what they termed *primary* and *secondary appraisal processes.* The former entail an initial evaluation as to whether some event is irrelevant to a perceiver, is relevant but not a threat, or is actually stressful. When an event or experience is seen as stressful, the secondary appraisal process performs a review of the individual's coping resources and available options for dealing with the stressor(s). How people appraise stressful situations can alter the impact such events or experiences have for them. To be sure, insider and outsider perspectives and interactions can shape whether a given encounter is pleasant and friendly or prejudicial and possibly discriminatory—or even ambiguous or ambivalent where attitudes are concerned (see, for example, Chapter 4 in Dunn, 2015). Moreover, appraisals can shift stress from being negative (a threat) to positive (a challenge); such positive reappraisals of stress can have both psychological and physiological benefits (Crum et al., 2020).

Most individuals assume that stress is harmful—that is, they adopt a *stress-is-debilitating mindset.* Other people, however, see stress as a favorable challenge, so they possess a *stress-is-enhancing mindset*, which affirms their abilities to deal with the stress effectively (Crum et al., 2017; Crum et al., 2021). Such perspectives would seem to be very helpful for examining how stress is processed when it is tied to disability, including the development and application of so-called wise interventions (e.g., Walton & Wilson, 2018; Wilson, 2011).

Finally, the appraisal of stress, while highly personal, can have other sources besides self-perception. Sources of potential stress can be found in the environment, as is the case for so-called ambient or environmental stress (e.g., excessive noise, traffic, pollution, crowding). Commuting to and from work can be stressful, for example, and experiencing negative affect might be compounded if the commuter also had a disability. Stress and related appraisals can also be influenced by a given culture and the resources that are available (or not) within it. The economic stress of disabled individuals is likely worsened when the cultures where they reside are plagued by unemployment, underemployment, educational challenges, and low wages or even poverty.

DIVERSITY, INTERSECTIONALITY, AND RESEARCH ISSUES

As we discussed in Chapter 2, disability is decidedly a form of diversity, though it is often not thought of as such in the popular mind. Yet we know that disabled people present a variety of other diverse qualities and demographic factors—everything from race to religion—that render them the largest minority group in the United States and perhaps around the globe (e.g., Perrin et al., 2019).

Awareness of diversity, equity, and inclusion issues is now a great concern of psychological scientists. A chief shortcoming of much of the research done in the 20th century and even early in the 21st century is the lack of representative participant samples. The bulk of the research studies done in the 1950s and 1960s, for example, relied primarily on college-aged White men as research participants. Eventually, college-aged women (mostly White), too, took part in research efforts at colleges and universities. Yet we know the data from such participants were likely influenced, perhaps even skewed, by the fact that most college students then (and to some extent now) hail from affluent, well-educated families that do not at all represent the normative qualities of the country's population (e.g., Bryant, 2021; Funder, 2024).

More to the point, some psychologists have characterized the participant samples typically used in mainstream psychological research as WEIRD (Henrich, 2021). In brief, Henrich and other researchers have pointed out that most participant samples are "WEIRD" because they only include people from westernized, educated, industrialized, rich, and democratic countries. In other words, such samples provide but one "slice"—and a narrow one at that—of the socio-cultural diversity to be found around the world (Heinrich et al., 2010; Syed, 2021). Should investigators in psychology and allied fields like cognitive science and behavioral economics be basing their theories and results on responses from such a limited group of people? Probably not, which means disciplines and the researcher-scholars within them need to redouble their efforts to recruit more diverse and representative samples for their work while also clearly acknowledging the shortcomings of current sampling procedures.

Minimally, producers and consumers of psychological research should worry about how and whether findings can be generalized to other people at other places and points in time. Generalizability is the degree to which the results of a given study can be applied to the understanding of other, broader contexts. If a sample is not representative of other larger groups, then we should not try to predict similar behavior within them, instead keeping our inferential focus to similar (WEIRD) groups, a choice that hampers knowledge.

In addition, traditional reliance on asking whether a respondent is "male or female" is probably too restricting an approach. This dichotomy fails to acknowledge the variety of genderqueer identities that now abound (Nestle et al., 2002). Indeed, it only creates another generalizability problem.

And what about disability and varieties of disabilities? It is often a challenge for rehabilitation psychologists to recruit enough disabled participants to take part in research studies. Why? Researchers can rarely promise that participation in any piece of research will necessarily improve the life or prognosis of the participants, which can limit their interest in taking part in the effort. Additionally, some participants may not be well enough to take part (e.g., those recently hospitalized or sent to rehab), just as others may not have the time or inclination to do so. These and other "qualifications" limit the sample sizes of research studies, which can reduce their statistical power, making discerning reliable effects a challenge.

Beyond recruiting challenges and sample size issues, sometimes care must be taken to identify participants who have similar disabilities. Why is this a challenge? It depends on the goals and scope of a given study. However, if a research effort is aimed at examining how people adapt to strokes, for example, shouldn't there be an attempt to recruit people who have had similar strokes (i.e., lesion locations within the brain) rather than accepting people with a variety of different stroke locations? Does such a difference matter? Researchers may not know until they verify whether it is (or is not) an issue. If you consider the wide variety of disabilities that affect people, the challenge of comparing even within a particular disability group can seem a bit daunting. Such a conclusion does not mean researchers should give up, but it does underscore the need to proceed with rigor and care to rule out threats to reliability, validity, and generalizability.

At the same time, researchers may want to consider taking part in open science initiatives where they preregister their study designs and procedures and then later share their data, analyses, and results so that other investigators can verify that their plans were ethically and scientifically sound (Appelbaum et al., 2018; Hong & Morgan, 2019). Given the challenges of recruiting disabled participants, using open science practices may be a way to develop research partnerships with colleagues that can expand participant recruitment while also fulfilling the goals of the foundational principles toward enhancing well-being among disabled people.

LANGUAGE FOR DISABILITY AND OTHER MINORITIZED COMMUNITIES

As was discussed in Chapter 2, the language used to describe disability, disabled people, and other minoritized groups has changed dramatically. Language evolves, a point that is also true for the terms used to refer to disability and people with disabilities. Person-first language has its place, but increasingly, identity-first language is championed by disabled persons (Andrews, 2020; Dunn & Andrews, 2015; see also Gernsbacher, 2017). Learning to use the language of disability is a way for professionals, including psychologists, to demonstrate cultural competence and to forge meaningful ties to disabled people and their families, communities, and allies. Arguably, the foundational principles speak to language advances through all seven principles, but especially the insider-outsider distinction (principle 2), adjustment to disability (principle 3), human dignity (principle 6), and advocacy (principle 7). No doubt, the language of and about disability will continue to change, and dedicated professionals—researchers, practitioners, and educators—can use the evolution of disability language to advance the foundational principles.

ACTIVISM AND ADVOCACY INCLINATIONS FOR CIVIL RIGHTS, HUMAN RIGHTS, AND GLOBAL HEALTH

The foundational principles (especially principle 7—advocacy efforts) can likely be used as material for rallying allies who want to advance the sociopolitical interests and well-being of the disability community. The Americans with Disabilities Act did change things for the better for disabled people in the United States, but this legislation did not create full parity between people with disabilities and their nondisabled peers. Profound educational, economic, and employment issues remain (Dunn, 2015). These and related structural factors in American society inhibit disabled people from fully participating and benefitting from opportunities that are more accessible for nondisabled individuals. Despite patriotic hyperbole and wishful thinking, upward social mobility remains elusive for many disabled persons. Indeed, disability is rarely characterized as a social class–related problem, but it might as well be one; less education leads to fewer options, including the problem of underemployment or even unemployment. Nor should it be forgotten that prejudicial attitudes and discriminatory hiring practices sometimes remain, social realities that prevent people with disabilities from achieving the livelihoods and lives they deserve.

Clearly, there are opportunities for disability allies to join forces with the disability community to protest and lobby against remaining inequalities. The foundational principles can be shared with interested advocates who want to better understand disability and the experience of disabled persons in the United States. As Henderson and Bryan (2011) observed, the human rights of some disabled persons have improved in the United States and in some other developed countries. However, the rights of individuals with more severe disabilities have not advanced as much as the rights of those with less severe disabilities. More to the point, we must remember that human rights are not the same thing as civil rights (Henderson & Bryan, 2011; see also Fleming, Roundtree, & Pierce, 2024).

Bentley and colleagues (2019b), too, highlight the role that the foundational principles play when applied to existing and rising disability-linked healthcare issues found around the world. These researchers suggest that when reinforced by theories based in social psychology, the foundational principles will help to empower disabled people and communities globally. According to Bentley et al., "Such insights are needed if equal human rights are to be truly realized by the world's most vulnerable populations, including individuals with disabilities in LMIC (low-and-middle-income countries) settings" (p. 74). Consideration of additional disability-related global health needs can be found in Bentley et al. (2019a)

Future Avenues of Inquiry for the Foundational Principles

As should be clear by now, the foundational principles of rehabilitation psychology are applicable to established topics tied to disability and the experience of disability. They should also be applicable to new areas of inquiry that either are active or are on the empirical horizon. In this section we first revisit a classic topic, the contact hypothesis, and then consider the opportunities afforded by research on culture change.

REVISITING THE CONTACT HYPOTHESIS

Allport (1954) argued that close, personal, and meaningful contact between members of different groups (i.e., majority group, minority group) could have favorable consequences for interpersonal relations. Hence, the *contact hypothesis* was born. As Gordon Allport wrote, prejudice

> may be reduced by equal status contact between majority and minority groups in the pursuit of common goals. The effect is greatly enhanced if this contact is sanctioned by institutional supports (i.e., by law, custom, or local atmosphere), and provided it is of a sort that leads to the perception of common interests and common humanity between members of the two groups (p. 281).

Pettigrew and Tropp (2006) published a detailed and influential meta-analysis of available intergroup contact studies that demonstrated that such contact "typically reduces prejudice," including the biases often found between disabled and nondisabled persons (see also Pettigrew et al, 2011).

Recently, Paluck et al. (2019) evaluated the "state of contact research from a policy perspective" (p. 129). To do so, these authors collected 27 published intergroup contact studies that relied on random assignment and delayed dependent measures in their research designs (close to two-thirds of these works appeared after the Pettigrew and Tropp [2006] article was published). Analysis of this expanded set of studies indicated that the earlier, general conclusion from Pettigrew and Tropp's work remains essentially valid.

However, Paluck et al.'s (2019) meta-analysis revealed that the contact effects do vary; indeed, intervention-oriented studies whose aims were to reduce racial or ethnic prejudices showed substantially weaker results than some others. Additionally, the investigators noted the absence of efforts focused on examining adults' racial or ethnic prejudices, a decided limitation for research tied to theory creation and policy implementation. Finally, Paluck and colleagues observed a lack of studies carefully investigating the key contact conditions recommended by Allport (1954) that should show when contact is most effective.

What about disability? Promoting meaningful contact between insiders and outsiders seems to be a useful approach for reducing negative feelings. Paluck et al.'s (2019) meta-analysis contained six studies involving disability (four involved individuals with intellectual disabilities, and the remaining two studies involved physical disabilities). The authors argued that prejudice aimed at people with intellectual or physical disabilities might differ from other types of prejudice due the ways disabled people are understood by nondisabled others (Fiske, 2011; see also Wu & Fiske, 2019). Of course, six studies are not many, and only one of them (on intellectual disabilities) involved adults over 25 years of age; the other studies used younger respondent samples. In addition, the updated contact hypothesis review, while favorably characterizing available research on disability, cannot inform us about a broader array of disabilities. In other words, there is much more work to be done, notably where designing and running controlled, randomized studies with varied samples of disability targets and delayed outcome measures are involved. One goal for readers interested in verifying the importance of Allport's contact hypothesis might be to design and conduct appropriate studies that incorporate ideas and perspectives grounded in the foundational principles.

We now turn to a larger issue: Can the dominant culture(s) in which disabled persons reside be changed so that they become more accepting of the differences represented by disability?

CALLS FOR CULTURE CHANGE

One of the main goals of the disability community and disability studies, as well as various disability activist groups (e.g., Not Dead Yet), has been to change our society's attitudes toward and understanding of disability as diversity and lived experience. In other words, these groups continue to try to create favorable cultural changes that

TABLE 10.1

Seven Principles Designed for Intentional Culture Change
Principle 1: People are culturally shaped shapers, so they can be culture changers.
Principle 2: Identifying, mapping, and evaluating the key levels of culture helps locate where to target change.
Principle 3: Culture change happens in both top-down and bottom-up ways and is more effective when the levels are all in alignment.
Principle 4: Culture change can be easier when it leverages existing core values and harder when it challenges deep-seated defaults and biases.
Principle 5: Culture change typically involves power struggles and identity threats.
Principle 6: Cultures interact with one another, and change can cause backlash, resistance, and clashes.
Principle 7: Timing and readiness matter.

Source: Hamedani et al. (2024)

advance the cause of disability rights and accompanying social justice issues (e.g., Trost et al., 2019). On the surface, such culture change would seem to be a daunting proposition. Yet research in social psychology suggests that changes in perceptions, attitudes, and behavior is possible (witness the previous discussion of the contact hypothesis, which has a modest but nonetheless sustained impact).

Hamedani and colleagues (2024) recently proposed seven principles for creating intentional culture change (see Table 10.1). To be sure, current American culture displays various social challenges that need to be addressed from a cultural change perspective (e.g., racism, sexism, LGBTQ+ rights, economic inequality, ageism), including social and civil rights for people with disabilities. Hamedani et al. (2024) propose a framework for what they call *intentional culture change* or approaches for thoughtfully promoting change by altering the mutually reinforcing qualities of a culture. These qualities include social and political policies, norms, practices, collective narratives, symbols, and goods and commodities, as well as attitudes, beliefs, and behaviors. Their arguments and methods are evidence-based—drawn from basic and applied research—and integrated. As the authors observed,

> As people work to change cultures across society, many everyday norms, practices, and policies are under scrutiny or in flux. From social protests over critical policy issues like access to abortion or voting rights; to shifting norms on sharing gender pronouns during personal introductions to speaking openly about mental health challenges in schools and workplaces; to

> changes to daily practices such as using reusable water bottles or commuting with an e-bike instead of a car, the spirit of culture change is all around. (p. 385)

Culture change, then, is in the air and the water, as it were. First, the COVID-19 pandemic and nascent climate change point to humanity's essential interdependence and the unsustainable nature of much of our modern existence (e.g., Nelson, 2022). Second, social movements aimed at addressing inequality—the MeToo and Black Lives Matter movements—fit here, as does activism focused on addressing ableism aimed at the disability community, among others. Third, dissatisfaction with governments and the tech industry only serve to highlight skepticism regarding who is serving whom. Shifting social norms tied to gender, sexuality, and work also suggest that change is happening. Technological advances illustrate the sheer power of the social world as well as the threats posed by artificial intelligence and undue influence of social media. Intentional culture change is now desired—that is, efforts to alter, modify, or improve a culture to benefit all its citizens.

In their article, Hamedani et al. (2024) address issues of social inequality and disparities in the United States; however, the principles they rely on (outlined in brief in Table 10.1) are readily applicable to other problems. One of their main points is important: Since people are culturally shaped "shapers," they, too, can change their cultures. The authors admit that few examples of large-scale change exist, but that should serve as the impetus to begin to enact intentional culture change, and the well-being and social standing of people with disabilities would seem to be an appropriate venue. The authors raise an important consideration, that culture change is unlikely to be built upon controlled lab work, online studies, or even computer simulations; rather, real culture change will rely on critical study of social change processes in field settings and natural settings in the real-world. Collaboration from relevant organizations and communities within the larger disability community will be essential.

Of course, there are some risks entailed in such approaches. Hamedani et al. (2024) warn readers that sociocultural change is "complex and multiply determined, and history is rife with the unintended consequences of human actions" (p. 14). To some extent, cultures evolve on their own without human design or intervention—people are essentially unaware of what is happening or why. Perhaps, then, humans must adapt to change simply because they have little or no control over it (Wilson, 2016; Wilson et al., 2014).

Nonetheless, Hamedani and colleagues (2024) highlight three reasons that potential culture change agents should accept the challenge:

- Change is an opportunity to strengthen cultures (in positive directions, via innovation and novelty).
- Change is an opportunity to cultivate imagination and speculation (exploring alternative futures or ways of being, perhaps developing new motivations on the way).
- Change is an opportunity to build (new norms, policies, practices, institutions, and organizations, as well as opportunities).

Although the source of such massive change is often collective unhappiness or distaste for the status quo, such social trends can promote space to reenvision, rethink, recreate, and redo society. Admittedly, this is a tall order, but one worthy of application of the foundational principles of rehabilitation psychology.

Only Connect: A Concluding Thought

> Only connect!
>
> —E. M. Forester (1910/1989, p. 195)

E. M. Forester was an English novelist. One of the themes explored in what is generally considered his most important novel, *Howards End* (Forester, 1989), is the human need or desire for *connection*. One type of connection is the ability to unite one's inner life (e.g., thoughts, feelings, identity) with the outer one (e.g., behavior, social life, other people). Forester observed that some people find it difficult to link their inner worlds with their outer, daily lives—often protecting the former from the latter. Others never learn to connect the two, and the resulting disconnection makes living difficult. Still others recognize that by connecting their inner lives with their outer existence they can make the most out of their lives; that is, they can live well and authentically.

I've often thought that this quote represents an overarching goal for the social psychology of disability and a particular forum wherein the foundational principles can operate: If only disabled and nondisabled people could truly connect with one another (see Dunn, 2019b). Disabled people want to connect with the wider social world while having their conditions accepted and perhaps understood. As outsiders, nondisabled people should welcome the opportunity to understand how insiders truly think, feel, and act, while also respecting and appreciating that disability is an important part of insider experiences—a neutral or even positive quality, not a burden. Perhaps the foundational principles can help insiders and outsiders connect better with one another. I hope that you will use the foundational principles to achieve this worthy end.

Precis and Prospects

The foundational principles represent a potentially primary focus for professionals and lay people who desire a framework for the science and practice of rehabilitation psychology. The principles have been both an implicit and now more explicit part of the field. They were linked to some of the field's important touchstones, including education and training issues, positive psychology, appraisal processes aligned with stress and coping, diversity and intersectionality research, language for disability and minority communities, and arenas for activism and advocacy. Two major areas of inquiry were identified for future application of the foundational principles—one classic (the contact hypothesis) and one new (intentional culture change). This final chapter concluded with a call for greater connection between insiders and outsiders.

THOUGHT QUESTIONS

1. Why should the foundational principles be considered a primary focus for professionals and lay people, as well as insiders and outsiders?
2. How can the foundational principles be made more explicit in rehabilitation psychology and the wider discipline of psychological science?
3. What is a foundational touchstone? Discuss one example from those presented in the chapter or, better yet, identify one of your own to add to the list.
4. How could the foundational principles be used to advance research efforts on the contact hypothesis as applied to disability and disabled people?
5. Why might the foundational principles be helpful where intentional culture change is concerned?
6. How can the foundational principles foster greater connection between insiders' and outsiders' inner and outer lives?

References

Ackerman, S., Zuroff, D. C., & Moskowitz, D. S. (2000). Generativity in midlife and young adults: Links to agency, communion, and subjective well-being. *International Journal of Aging & Human Development, 50*, 17–41.

Aguinis, H. (1993). Action research and scientific method: Presumed discrepancies and actual similarities. *Journal of Applied Behavioral Science 29*(4), 416–431.

Allport, G. W. (1954). *The nature of prejudice*. Addison-Wesley.

Altman, B. (2001). Disability definitions, models, classification schemes, and applications. In G. Albrecht, K. Seelman, & M. Bury (Eds.), *Handbook of disability studies* (pp. 97–122). Sage.

American Board of Professional Psychology/American Board of Rehabilitation Psychology. (2022). *Certification guidelines and procedures: Candidate's manual.* Retrieved April 8, 2019, from https://abpp.org/wp-content/uploads/2022/10/ABRPCandidateManual-Adopted9June2022.pdf

American Educational Research Association, American Psychological Association, National Council on Measurement in Education & Joint Committee on Standards for Educational and Psychological Testing. (2014). *Standards for educational and psychological testing*. American Educational Research Association.

American Psychological Association (APA). (2017). *Multicultural guidelines: An ecological approach to context, identity, and intersectionality*. https://www.apa.org/about/policy/multucultural-guidelines.pdf

American Psychological Association. (2019). *APA resolution on support of universal design and accessibility in education, training, and practice*. Author.

American Psychological Association. (2020). *Publication manual of the American Psychological Association* (7th ed.).

American Psychological Association (APA). (2021). *Equity, diversity, and inclusion framework*. file:///Users/medsd01/Documents/Foundational%20Principles%20Book/Chapter%202/APA%20EDI.pdf

American Psychological Association. (2023). *Equity, diversity, and inclusion: Inclusive language guide* (2nd ed). https://www.apa.org/about/apa/equity-diversity-inclusion/language-guidelines.pdf
American Psychological Association. (2024a). *APA Dictionary*. https://dictionary.apa.org/self
American Psychological Association. (2024b). *Equity, diversity, and inclusion*. https://www.apa.org/topics/equity-diversity-inclusion
Americans with Disabilities Act of 1990, Pub. L. No. 101-336, 104 Stat. 327 (1991).
Americans with Disabilities Act of 1990, Pub. L. No. 101-336, 104 Stat. 328 (1990).
Anderson, K. J. (2010). *Benign bigotry: The psychology of subtle prejudice*. Cambridge University Press.
Andrews, E. A. (2020). *Disability as diversity: Developing cultural competence*. Oxford University Press.
Andrews, E. A., Ayers., K. B., Brown, K. S., Dunn, D. S., & Pilarski, C. (2021). No body is expendable: Medical rationing and disability justice during the Covid-19 pandemic. *American Psychologist, 76*(3), 751–761. http://doi.org/10.1037/amp0000709
Andrews, E. E. (2017). Disability models. In M. A. Budd, S. Hough, S. T. Wegener, & W. Stiers (Eds.), *Practical psychology in medical rehabilitation*. (pp. 77–83). Springer International Publishing; Springer Nature.
Andrews, E. E. (2020). *Disability as diversity: Developing cultural competence*. Oxford University Press.
Andrews, E. E., Ayers, K., Dunn, D. S., & Wehmeyer, M. L. (Eds.). (in press). *Oxford handbook of positive psychology and disability* (2nd ed.). Oxford University Press.
Andrews, E. E., Forber-Pratt, A. J., Mona, L. R., Lund, E. M., Pilarski, C. R., & Balter, R. (2019). #SaytheWord: A disability culture commentary on the erasure of "disability." *Rehabilitation Psychology, 64*(2), 111–118. http://doi.org/10.1037/rep0000258
Andrews, E. E., Kuemmel, A., Williams, J., Pilarski, C. R., Dunn, M., & Lund, E. M. (2013). Providing culturally competent supervision to trainees with disabilities in rehabilitation settings. *Rehabilitation Psychology, 58*(3), 233–244. http://doi.org/10.1037/a0033338
Andrews, E. E., Pilarski, C. R., Ayers, K., & Dunn, D. S. (2023). Advocacy: The seventh foundational principle and core competency of rehabilitation psychology. *Rehabilitation Psychology, 68*(2), 103–111. http://doi.org/10.1037/rep0000492
Andrews, E. E., Powell, R. M., & Ayers, K. (2022). The evolution of disability language: Choosing terms to describe disability. *Disability and Health Journal*. http://doi.org/10.1016/j.dhjo.2022.101328
Antonak, R. F. (1981). Psychometric analysis of the Attitude Toward Disabled Persons Scale, Form-O. *Rehabilitation Counseling Bulletin, 23*, 169–176.
Antonak, R. F., & Livneh, H. (1988). *Measurement of attitudes toward people with disabilities: Methods, psychometrics, and scales*. Charles C. Thomas.
Antonovsky, A. (1987). *Unravelling the mystery of health: How people manage stress and stay well*. Jossey-Bass.
Appelbaum, M., Cooper, H., Kline, R. B., Mayo-Wilson, E., Nezu, A. M., & Rao, S. M. (2018). Journal article reporting standards for quantitative research in psychology: The APA Publications and Communications Board task force report. *American Psychologist, 73*, 3–25.
Aristotle. (1984). *Complete works: Revised Oxford translation in 2 volumes* (J. Barnes, Ed.). Princeton University Press.
Aronson, J., Lustina, M. J., Good, C., Keough, K., Steele, C. M., & Brown, J. (1999). White men can't do math: Necessary and sufficient factors in stereotype threat. *Journal of Experimental Social Psychology, 35*, 29–46. http://doi.org/10.1006/jesp.1998.1371
Asch, A. (1988). Disability: Its place in the psychology curriculum. In P. Bronstein & K. Quinn (Eds.), *Teaching a psychology of people: Resources for gender and socio-cultural awareness* (pp. 156–167). American Psychological Association. http://doi.org/10.1037/10066-019
Asch, S. E. (1946). Forming impressions of personality. *Journal of Abnormal and Social Psychology, 41*, 258–290. http://doi.org/10.1037/h0055756
Aspinwall, L. G., & Staudinger, U. M. (Eds.). (2003). *A psychology of human strengths: Fundamental questions and future directions for a positive psychology*. American Psychological Association.
Audi, R. (Ed.). (1995). *The Cambridge dictionary of philosophy*. Cambridge University Press.

Banaji, M. R., & Heiphetz, L. (2010). Attitudes. In S. T. Fiske, D. Gilbert, & G. Lindzey (Eds.), *Handbook of social psychology* (5th ed., Vol. 1, pp. 353–393). Wiley.

Bandler, R. J., Jr., Madaras, G. R., & Bem, D. J. (1968). Self-observation as a source of pain perception. *Journal of Personality and Social Psychology, 9*(3), 205–209.

Banyard, P., & Hulme, J. A. (2015). Giving psychology away: How George Miller's vision is being realised by psychological literacy. *Psychology Teaching Review, 21*(2), 93–101.

Bargh, J. A., Chaiken, S., Raymond, P., & Hymes, C. (1996). The automatic evaluation effect: Unconditional automatic attitude activation with a pronunciation task. *Journal of Experimental Social Psychology, 32*, 104–128. http://doi.org/10.1006/jesp.1996.0005

Barker, R. G. (1947). The somatopsychologic problem. *Psychosomatic Medicine, 9*, 192–196.

Barker, R. G. (1960). Foreword. In B. A. Wright, *Physical disability: A psychological approach* (pp. xiii–xv). Harper & Row.

Barker, R. G., Wright, B. A., Myerson, L., & Gonick, M. R. (1953). *Adjustment to physical handicap and illness: A survey of the social psychology of physique and disability* (2nd ed., Bulletin 55). Social Science Research Council Bulletin.

Bat-Chava, Y. (1994). Group identification and self-esteem of deaf adults. *Personality and Social Psychology Bulletin, 20*(5), 494–502. http://doi.org/10.1177/0146167294205006

Bauer, J. J. (2021). *The transformative self: Personal growth, narrative identity, and the good life*. Oxford University Press. http://doi.org/10.1080/17439760.2013.830764

Bauman, D., & Murray, J. J. (2014, November 13). An introduction to Deaf Gain: Shifting our perceptions of Deaf people from hearing loss to deaf gain. *Deaf Gain*. https://www.psychologytoday.com/us/blog/deaf-gain/201411/introduction-deaf-gain

Baumeister, R. F., & Bushman, B. J. (2014). *Social psychology and human nature*. Cengage.

Baumeister, R. F., Bratlavsky, E., Finkenauer, C., & Vohs, K. D. (2001). Bad is stronger than good. *Review of General Psychology, 5*, 323–370. http://doi.org/10.1037/1089-2680.5.4.323

Baumeister, R. F., & Vohs, K. D. (2002). The pursuit of meaningfulness in life. In C. R. Snyder & S. J. Lopez (Eds.), *Handbook of positive psychology* (pp. 608–618). Oxford University Press.

Baumeister, R. F., Vohs, K. D., Aaker, J. L., & Garbinsky, E. N. (2013). Some key differences between a happy life and a meaningful life. *Journal of Positive Psychology, 8*(6), 505–516.

Bem, D. J. (1967). Self-perception: An alternative interpretation of cognitive dissonance phenomena. *Psychological Review, 74*(3), 183–200.

Bem, D. J. (1972). Self-perception theory. In L. Berkowitz (Ed.), *Advances in experimental social psychology* (Vol. 6, pp. 1–62). Academic Press.

Bentley, J., MacLachlan, M., Geiser, P., Mannan, H., & Zou, H. (2019a). Disability-related global health needs. In L. A., Brenner, S. A. Reid-Arndt, T. R. Elliott, R. G. Frank, & B. Caplan (Eds.), *Handbook of rehabilitation psychology* (3rd ed., pp. 443–455). American Psychological Association. https://doi.org/10/1037/0000129-026

Bentley, J. A., Tingey, J. L., Lum, J., & Ho, S.-E. (2019b). Rehabilitation psychology's foundational principles and social psychological theories: Intersections and applications in global health. In D. S. Dunn (Ed.), *Understanding the experience of disability: Perspectives from social and rehabilitation psychology* (pp. 74–89). Oxford University Press.

Berger, M. W. (2023, March 6). Does more money correlate with greater happiness? *Penn Today.* https://penntoday.upenn.edu/news/does-more-money-correlate-greater-happiness-Penn-Princeton-research

Berghs, M. J., Atkin, K. M., Graham, H. M., Hatton, C., & Thomas, C. (2016). Implications for public health research of models and theories of disability: A scoping study and evidence synthesis. *Public Health Research, 4*(8). http://doi.org/10.3310/phr04080

Bergink, J. (2015). Happiness: Its' not just your genes, stupid! [Weblog post]. http://www.forastateofhappiness.com/tag/50-10-40-formula/

Berne, P., Morales, A. L., Langstaff, D., & Invalid, S. (2018). Ten principles of disability justice. *WSQ: Women's Study Quarterly, 46*(1–2), 227–230. https://doi.org/10.1353/wsq.2018.0003

Bhattarai, J., Bentley, J., Morean, W., Wegener, S. T., & Pollack Porter, K. M. (2020). Promoting equity at the population level: Putting the foundational principles into practice through disability advocacy. *Rehabilitation Psychology, 65*(2), 87–100. https://doi.org/10.1037/rep0000321

Bishop, M., Huang, Y. (J.), Zhou, K., & Baumunk, M. (2024). Quality of life and psychosocial adaptation to chronic illness and disability. In I. Marini, A. R. Fleming, & M. Bishop (Eds.), *The psychological and social impact of chronic illness and disability* (pp. 215–232). Springer Publishing.

Biswas-Diener, R. (2013, April 6). One myth of positive psychology clearly explained: How science is spun into myth. *Psychology Today*. http://www.psychologytoday.com/blog/significant-results/201304/one-myth-positive-psychology-clearly-explained

Blair, T., & Minkler, M. (2009). Participatory action research with older adults: Key principles in practice. *The Gerontologist, 49*(5), 651–662. https://doi.org/10.1093/geront/gnp049

Bloom, P. (2010). *How pleasure works: The new science of why we like what we like*. Norton.

Bodenhamer, E., Achterberg-Lawlis, J., Kevorkian, G., Belanus, A., & Cofer, J. (1983). Staff and patient perceptions of the psychosocial concerns of spinal cord injured persons. *American Journal of Physical Medicine, 62*, 182–193.

Bogart, K. R. (2014). The role of disability self-concept in adaptation to congenital or acquired disability. *Rehabilitation Psychology, 59*, 107–115. http://doi.org/10.1037/a0031691

Bogart, K. R., & Dunn, D. S. (2019a). Ableism: Special issue introduction. *Journal of Social Issues, 75*, 650–664.

Bogart, K. R., & Dunn, D. S. (Eds.). (2019b). Ableism. *Journal of Social Issues, 75*(3), 643–984.

Bogart, K. R., Lund, E. M., & Rottenstein, A. (2018). Disability pride protects self-esteem through the rejection-identification model. *Rehabilitation Psychology, 63*(1), 155–159. https://doi.org/10.1037/rep0000166

Bogart, K. R., & Nario-Redman, M. R. (2019). An exploration of disability self-categorization, identity, and pride. In D. S. Dunn (Ed.), *Understanding the experience of disability: Perspectives from social and rehabilitation psychology* (pp. 252–267). Oxford University Press.

Boldry, J. G., Gaertner, L., & Quinn, J. (2007). Measuring the measures: A meta-analytic investigation of outgroup homogeneity. *Group Processes & Intergroup Relations, 10*, 157–178. http://doi.org/10.1177/1368430207075153

Bolt, M. A., & Dunn, D. S. (2016). *Pursuing human strengths: A positive psychology guide* (2nd ed.). Worth.

Bonanno, G. A. (2012). Uses and abuses of the resilience construct: Loss, trauma, and health-related adversities. *Social Science & Medicine, 74*, 753–756. http://doi.org/10.1016/j.socscimed.2011.11.022

Bonanno, G. A., & Diminich, E. D. (2013). Annual research review: Positive adjustment to adversity—trajectories of minimal-impact resilience and emergent resilience. *The Journal of Child Psychology and Psychiatry, 54*(4), 378–401. http://doi.org/10.1111/jcpp.12021

Bowleg, L. (2012). The problem with the phrase *women and minorities*: Intersectionality—an important theoretical framework for public health. *American Journal of Public Health, 102*(7), 1267–1273. http://doi.org/10.2105/AJPH.2012.300750

Boyd, N. F., Sutherland, H. J., Heasman, K. Z., Trichler, D. L., & Cummings, B. J. (1990). Whose utilities for decision analysis? *Medical Decision Making, 10*, 58–67. http://doi.org/10.1177/0272989X.66.6.979

Breckler, S. J. (1984). Empirical validation of affect, behavior, and cognition as distinct components of attitude. *Journal of Personality and Social Psychology, 37*, 917–927.

Brehm, S. S., & Brehm, J. W. (1981). *Psychological reactance*. Wiley.

Brenner, L. A., Reid-Arndt, S. A., Elliott, T. R., Frank, R. G., & Caplan, B. (Eds.). (2019). *Handbook of rehabilitation psychology* (3rd ed.). American Psychological Association.

Brewer, M. B., & Brown, R. J. (1998). Intergroup relations. In D. T. Gilbert, S. T. Fiske, & G. Lindzey (Eds.), *The handbook of social psychology* (4th ed., Vol. 2). McGraw-Hill.

Brickman, P., & Campbell, D. T. (1971). Hedonic relativism and planning the good society. In M. H. Appley (Ed.), *Adaptation level theory: A symposium* (pp. 287–302). Academic Press.

Brickman, P., Coates, D., & Janoff-Bulman, R. (1978). Lottery winners and accident victims: Is happiness relative? *Journal of Personality and Social Psychology, 36*(8), 917–927. http://doi.org/10.1037/0022-3514.36.8.917

Brody, H. (2012). From an ethics of rationing to an ethics of waste avoidance. *The New England Journal of Medicine, 366*, 1949–1951. http://doi.org/10.1056/NEJMp1203365

Brown, N. J. L., & Rohrer, J. M. (2019). Easy as (happiness) pie? A critical evaluation of a popular model of the determinants of well-being. *Journal of Happiness Studies: An Interdisciplinary Forum on Subjective Well-Being, 21*(4), 1285–1301. http://doi.org/10.1007/s10902-019-00128-4

Brueggemann, B. J. (2013). Disabilities studies/disability culture. In M. L. Wehmeyer (Ed.), *Oxford handbook of positive psychology and disability* (pp. 279–299). Oxford University Press.

Bruyère, S. M., & Peterson, D. B. (2005). Introduction to the special section on the International Classification of Functioning, Disability, and Health (ICF): Implications for rehabilitation psychology. *Rehabilitation Psychology, 50*, 103–104. doi: 10.1037/0090-5550.50.2.103

Bryant, F. B., & Veroff, J. (2007). *Savoring: A new model of positive experience*. Erlbaum.

Bryant, J. (2021, May 10). Percentages of Americans with a college degree. Best Colleges. https://www.bestcolleges.com/news/analysis/2021/07/01/how-many-americans-have-college-degrees

Bryant, J. (2023, May 10). *Percentage of Americans with a college degree*. Best Colleges. https://www.bestcolleges.com/news/analysis/2021/07/01/how-many-americans-have-college-degrees

Burkhead, E. J., Deborah, J., & Marini, I. (1996). Humor, coping, and adaptation to disability. *Journal of Applied Rehabilitation Counseling, 27*, 50–53.

Caldwell, J. (2011). Disability identity of leaders in the self-advocacy movement. *Intellectual and Developmental Disabilities, 49*, 316–346. http://doi.org/10.1352/1934-9556

Callahan C. (2004). Facial disfigurement and sense of self in head and neck cancer. *Social Work in Health Care. 40*(2), 73–87. http://doi.org/10.1300/j010v40n02_05.

Campbell, F. (2001). Inciting legal fictions: 'Disability's' date with ontology and the ableist body of the law. *Griffith Law Review, 10*(1), 42–62.

Cassell, C., & Johnson, P. (2006). Action research: Explaining the diversity. *Human Relations 54*(6), 783–814. http://doi.org/10.1177/0018726706067080

CDC. (2022, May 18). Disability and Health Data System (DHDS). Centers for Disease Control and Prevention. https://www.cdc.gov/ncbddd/disabilityandhealth/dhds/index.html

Chan, F., Gelman, J. S., Ditchman, N., Kim, J.-H., & Chiu, C.-Y. (2009). The World Health Organization ICF model as a conceptual framework of disability. In F. Chan, E. Da Silva Cardoso, & J. A. Chronister (Eds.), *Understanding psychosocial adjustment to chronic illness and disability: A handbook for evidence-based practitioners in rehabilitation* (pp. 23–50). Springer.

Chan, C. C., Lee, T. M. C., Yuen, H. K., & Chan, F. (2002). Attitudes towards people with disabilities between Chinese rehabilitation and business students: An implication for practice. *Rehabilitation Psychology, 47*, 324–338. http://doi.org/10.1037/0090-5550.47.3.324

Chan, F., Livneh, H., Pruett, S., Wang, C.-C., & Zheng, L. X. (2009). Societal attitudes toward disability: Concepts, measurements, and interventions. In F. Chan, E. da Silva, & J. A. Chronister (Eds.), *Understanding psychosocial adjustment to chronic illness and disability: A handbook for evidence-based practitioners in rehabilitation* (pp. 333–367). Springer.

Chan, F., da Silva Cordoso, E., & Chronister, J. A. (Eds.). (2009). *Understanding psychosocial adjustment to chronic illness and disability: A handbook for evidence-based practitioners in rehabilitation*. Springer.

Charmaz, K. (1994). Identity dilemmas of chronically ill men. *Sociological Quarterly, 35*(2), 269–288. http://doi.org/10.1111/j.1533-8525.1994.tb00410.x

Charmaz, K. (1995). The body, identity, and self. *Sociological Quarterly*, *36*(4), 657–680. http://doi.org/10.1111/j.1533-8525.1995.tb00459.x

Chen, A., Ahmad, M., Flescher, A., Freeman, W. L., Little, S., Martins, P. N., Veatch, R. M., Wightman, A., & Ladin, K. (2020). Access to transplantation for persons with intellectual disability: Strategies for nondiscrimination. *American Journal of Transplantation*. *20*(8), 2009–2016. http://doi.org/10.1111/ajt.15755

Chen, R. K., Brodwin, M. G., Cardoso, E., & Chan, F. (2002). Attitudes towards people with disabilities in the social context of dating and marriage: A comparison of American, Taiwanese and Singaporean college students. *Journal of Rehabilitation*, *68*, 5–11.

Cheng, S., Mendoza, S. A., Ng, L. C., Nittrouer, C. L., & Hebl, M. (2019). Disability in the workplace. In D. S. Dunn (Ed.), *Understanding the experience of disability: Perspectives from social ad rehabilitation psychology* (pp. 223–238). Oxford University Press.

Collins, R. L., Taylor, S. E., & Skokan, L. A. (1990). A better world or a shattered vision? Changes in life perspective following victimization. *Social Cognition*, *8*, 263–285. http://doi.org/10.1521/soco.1990.8.3.263

Compton, W. C. (2004). *An introduction to positive psychology*. Thompson-Wadsworth.

Conder, J., Milner, P., & Mirfin-Veitch, B. (2011). Reflections on a participatory project: The rewards and challenges for the lead researchers. *Journal of Intellectual and Developmental Disability*, *36*(1), 39–48. http://doi.org/10.3109/13668250.2010.548753

Cooper Jones, C. (2022). *Easy beauty: A memoir*. Avid Reader Press.

Corrigan, P. W. (Ed.). (2014). *The stigma of disease and disability: Understanding causes and overcoming injustices*. American Psychological Association. http://doi.org/10.1037/14297-000.

Corrigan, P. W., River, L. P., Lundin, R. K., Uphoff Wasowski, K., Campion, J., Mathisen, J., Goldstein, H., Bergman, M., Gagnon, C., & Kubiak, M. A. (2000). Stigmatizing attributions about mental illness. *Journal of Community Psychology*, *28*(1), 91–102. http://doi.org/10.1002/(SICI)1520-6629(200001)28:1<91::AIJCOP9>3.0.CO;2-M

Corrigan, P. W., & Watson, A. C. (2002). Understanding the impact of stigma on people with mental illness. *World Psychiatry*, *1*(1), 16–20.

Cox, D. R., Cox, R. H., & Caplan, B. (2013). *Consumer protection. Specialty competencies in rehabilitation psychology* (pp. 101–106). Oxford University Press. https://doi.org/10.1093/med:psych/9780195389241.003.0008

Craig, A. (2012). Resilience in people with physical disabilities. In P. Kennedy (Ed.), *Oxford handbook of rehabilitation psychology* (pp. 474–491). Oxford University Press. https://doi.org/10.1093/oxfordhb/9780199733989.013.0026

Craig, E. (Ed.) (1998a). *Routledge encyclopedia of philosophy* (Vol. 3). Routledge.

Craig, E. (Ed.) (1998b). *Routledge encyclopedia of philosophy* (Vol. 4). Routledge.

Crenshaw, K. (1989). Demarginalizing the intersection of race and sex: A Black feminist critique of antidiscrimination doctrine and antiracist politics. *The University of Chicago Legal Forum*, 1989 (1), 139–167. https://chicagobound.uchicago.edu/uclf/vol1989/iss1/8/

Crum, A. J., Akinola, M., Martin, A., & Fath, S. (2017). The role of stress mindset in shaping cognitive, emotional, and physiological responses to challenging and threatening stress. *Anxiety, Stress, and Coping*, *30*(4), 379–395. https://doi.org/10.1080/10615806.1275585

Crum, A. J., Handley, M. I. J., & Smith, E. N. (2021). The stress-mindset intervention. In G. M. Walton & A. J. Crum (Eds.), *Handbook of wise interventions: How social psychology can help people change* (pp. 217–238). The Guilford Press.

Crum, A. J., Jamieson, J. P., & Akinola, M. (2020). Optimizing stress: An integrated intervention for regulating stress responses. *Emotion*, *20*(1), 120–125. https://doi.org/10.1037/emo0000670.supp

Csikszentmihalyi, M. (1997). *Finding flow*. Basic Books.

Csikszentmihalyi, M. (2006). Introduction. In M. Csikszentmihalyi & I. S. Csikszentmihalyi (Eds.), *A life worth living: Contributions to positive psychology* (pp. 3–14). Oxford University Press.

Csikszentmihalyi, M. (2021). Flow: A component of the good life. In A. Kostić & D. Chadee (Eds.), *Positive psychology: An international perspective* (pp. 193–200). Wiley Blackwell.

Cuddy, A. J. C., Fiske, S. T., & Glick, P. (2007). The BIAS map: Behaviors from inter-group affect and stereotypes. *Journal of Personality and Social Psychology, 92*, 631–648. https://doi.org/10.1037/0022-3514.92.4.631

Cuddy, A. J. C., Fiske, S. T., & Glick, P. (2008). Warmth and competence as universal dimensions of social perception: The stereotype content model and the BIAS map. In M. P. Zanna (Ed.), *Advances in experimental social psychology* (Vol. 40, pp. 61–149). Academic Press.

Darling, R. B. (2013). *Disability and identity: Negotiating self in a changing society*. Boulder, CO: Lynne Rienner Publishers.

Darling, R. B., & Heckert, D. A. (2010). Orientation toward disability: Differences over the lifecourse. *International Journal of Disability, Development, and Education, 57*, 131–143. https://doi.org/10.1080/10349121003750489

Davis, L. J. (Ed.). (2013). *The disability studies reader* (4th ed.). Routledge.

Deal, M. (2003). Disabled people's attitudes toward other impairment groups: A hierarchy of impairments. *Disability & Society, 18*(7), 897–910. https://doi.org/10.1080/0968759032000127317

Deci, E. L., & Ryan, R. M. (2000). The support of autonomy and the control of behavior. In E. T. Higgins & A. W. Kruglanski (Eds.), *Motivational science: Social and personality perspectives*. (pp. 128–145). Psychology Press.

Dembo, T. (1964). Sensitivity of one person to another. *Rehabilitation Literature, 25*, 231–235.

Dembo, T. (1970). The utilization of psychological knowledge in rehabilitation. *Welfare Review, 8*, 1–7.

Dembo, T. (1982). Some problems in rehabilitation as seen by a Lewinian. *Journal of Social Issues, 38*, 133–139. https://doi.org/10.1111/j.1540-4560.1982.tb00848.x

Dembo, T., Leviton, G. L., & Wright, B. A. (1956). Adjustment to misfortune: A problem of social-psychological rehabilitation. *Artificial Limbs, 3*(2), 4–62.0

de Montaigne, M. (1991). *The complete essays* (M. A. Screech, Trans.). Penguin. (Original work published 1580)

DePape, A. M., & Lindsay, S. (2015). Lived experiences from the perspective of individuals with autism spectrum disorder: A qualitative meta-analysis. *Focus on Autism and Other Developmental Disabilities, 31*(1), 60–71. https://doi.org/10.1177/1088357615587504

DePaulo, B. M. (2015). *Marriage vs. single life: How science and the media got it so wrong*. CreateSpace.

DePaulo, B. M. (2018). Toward a positive psychology of single life. In D. S. Dunn (Ed.), *Positive psychology: Established and emerging issues* (pp. 251–275). Routledge.

Diener, E., & Diener, C. (1996). Most people are happy. *Psychological Science, 7*, 181–185.

Diener, E., Fraser, S. C., Beaman, A. L., & Kelem, R. T. (1976). Effects of deindividuation variables on stealing among Halloween trick-or-treaters. *Journal of Personality and Social Psychology, 33*, 178–183. https://doi.org/10.1037/0022-3514.33.2.178

Diener, E., Lucas, R. E., & Scollon, C. N. (2006). Beyond the hedonic treadmill: Revising the adaptation theory of well-being. *American Psychologist, 61*, 305–314. https://doi.org/10.1037/0003-066X.61.4.305

Diener, E., & Seligman, M. E. P. (2002). Very happy people. *Psychological Science, 13*, 80–83.

Diener, E., Suh, E. M., Lucas, R. E., & Smith, H. L. (1999). Subjective well-being: Three decades of progress. *Psychological Bulletin, 125*, 276–302.

Di Giulio, G. (2003). Sexuality and people living with physical or developmental disabilities: A review of key issues. *Canadian Journal of Human Sexuality, 12*(1), 53–68.

Dijkers, M. (1997). Quality of life after spinal cord injury: A meta-analysis of the effects of the disablement components. *Spinal Cord, 35*, 829–840. https://doi.org/10.1037/0033-2909.125.2.276

Dijkers, M., & Cushman, L. A. (1990). Differences between rehabilitation disciplines in views of depression in spinal cord injury patients. *Paraplegia, 28*, 380–391. https://doi.org/10.1038/sc.1990.51

Dijkers, M. P. J. M. (2005). Quality of life of individuals with a spinal cord injury: A review of conceptualization, measurement, and research findings. *Journal of Rehabilitation Research and Development*, *42*, 87–110. https://doi.org/10.1682/JRRD.2004.08.0100

Dion, K. K., Berscheid, E., & Walster, E. (1972). What is beautiful is good. *Journal of Personality and Social Psychology*, *24*, 285–290. https://doi.org/10.1037/h0033731

Division 22. (2024). *Rehabilitation psychology*. https://www.div22.org/

Dixon-Ibarra, A., Catena, M., and Krahn, G. (2019). Epidemiology of disability and health. In L. A. Brenner, S. A. Reid-Arndt, T. R. Elliott, R. G. Frank, & B. Caplan, (Eds.). *Handbook of rehabilitation psychology* (3rd ed., pp. 125–142). American Psychological Association. http://doi.org/10.1037/0000129-009

Dovidio, J. F., & Fiske, S. T. (2012). Under the radar: How unexamined biases in decision-making processes in clinical interactions can contribute to healthcare disparities. *American Journal of Public Health*, *102*(5), 945–952.

Dovidio, J. F., Major, B., & Crocker, J. (2000). Stigma: Introduction and overview. In T. F. Heatherton, R. E. Kleck, M. R. Hebl, & J. G. Hull (Eds.), *The social psychology of stigma* (p. 1–28). Guilford.

Dovidio, J. F., Pagotto, L., & Hebl, M. R. (2011). Implicit attitudes and discrimination against people with disabilities. In R. L. Wiener & S. L. Willborn (Eds.), *Disability and age discrimination: Perspectives in law and psychology* (pp. 157–183). Springer. http://doi.org/10.1007/978-1-4419-6293-5_9

Duggan, C. H., & Dijkers, M. (2001). Quality of life after spinal cord injury: A qualitative analysis. *Rehabilitation Psychology*, *46*, 3–27. http://doi.org/10.1037/0090-5550.46.1.3

Dunn, D. S. (1996). Well-being following amputation: Salutary effects of positive meaning, optimism, and control. *Rehabilitation Psychology*, *41*, 285–302. http://doi.org/10.1037/0090-5550.41.4.285

Dunn, D. S. (2009). Teaching about disability: Cultures of experience, not expectation. In R. A. R. Gurung & L. Prieto (Eds.), *Got culture? Best practices for incorporating culture into the* curriculum (pp. 101–114). Stylus.

Dunn, D. S. (2015). *The social psychology of disability*. Oxford University Press.

Dunn, D. S. (2016). Teaching about psychosocial aspects of disability: Emphasizing the person-environment relation. *Teaching of Psychology*, *43*, 255–262.

Dunn, D. S. (2018). A positive psychology for disability and rehabilitation: Recent advances. In D. S. Dunn (Ed.), *Positive psychology: Established and emerging issues* (pp. 236–250). Taylor & Francis.

Dunn, D. S. (2019a). Judging disability: Some biases identified by social psychology and rehabilitation psychology. In D. S. Dunn (Ed.), *Understanding the experience of disability: Perspectives from social and rehabilitation psychology* (pp. 24–38). Oxford University Press.

Dunn, D. S. (2019b). Only connect: The social psychology of disability. In L. A. Brenner, S. Reid-Arndt, T. R. Elliott, R. G. Frank, & B. Caplan (Eds.), *Handbook of rehabilitation psychology* (3rd ed., pp. 143–156). American Psychological Association.

Dunn, D. S. (2019c). Outsider privileges can lead to insider disadvantages: Some psychosocial aspects of ableism. *Journal of Social Issues*, *75*, 665–685.

Dunn, D. S. (Ed.). (2019d). *Understanding the experience of disability: Perspectives from social and rehabilitation psychology*. Oxford University Press.

Dunn, D. S. (2022). Resilience, disability, and intrapersonal factors viewed through the lens of rehabilitation psychology's foundational principles. In M. L. Wehmeyer & D. S. Dunn (Eds.), *The positive psychology of personal factors: Implications for understanding disability* (pp. 127–146). Lexington Books; Rowman & Littlefield.

Dunn, D. S. (2024). Recognizing, understanding, and constructively responding to ableism. In I. Marini, A. R. Fleming, & M. Bishop (Eds.), *The psychological and social impact of illness and disability* (8th ed.) (pp. 69–83). Springer Publishing.

Dunn, D. S., & Andrews, E. (2015). Person-first and identity-first language: Developing psychologists' cultural competence using disability language. *American Psychologist, 70*, 255–264.

Dunn, D. S., & Ayers, K. (in press). Resilience, problem solving, and the experience of disability: A positive psychological perspective. In E. E. Andrews, K. Ayers, D. S. Dunn, & M. L. Wehmeyer (Eds)., *The Oxford Handbook of Positive Psychology and Disability*. Oxford University Press.

Dunn, D. S., & Brody, C. (2008). Defining the good life following acquired physical disability. *Rehabilitation Psychology, 53*, 413–425.

Dunn, D. S., Brown, K., Forber-Pratt, A., Gorgens, K., Gray, A., Rohe, D., Tackett, M. J., & Wilson, C. (2021, February). Foundational principles: Responding to the crises of our time. Town hall panel at the annual conference on Rehabilitation Psychology 2021 [virtual conference].

Dunn, D. S., & Burcaw, S. (2013), Disability identity: Exploring narratives accounts of disability. *Rehabilitation Psychology, 58*(2), 148–157. http://doi.org/10.1037/a0031691

Dunn, D. S., & Dougherty, S. B. (2005). Prospects for a positive psychology of rehabilitation. *Rehabilitation Psychology, 50*, 305–311.

Dunn, D. S., Ehde, D. M., & Wegener, S. T. (2016). The foundational principles as psychological lodestars: Theoretical inspiration and empirical direction in rehabilitation psychology. *Rehabilitation Psychology, 61*(1), 1–6. http://doi.org/10.1037/rep0000082

Dunn, D. S., & Elliott, T. R. (2005). Revisiting a constructive classic: Wright's *Physical Disability: A Psychosocial Approach. Rehabilitation Psychology, 50*, 183–189.

Dunn, D. S., & Elliott, T. R. (2008). The place and promise of theory in rehabilitation psychology research. *Rehabilitation Psychology, 53*, 254–267.

Dunn, D. S., Fisher, D. J., & Beard, B. M. (2012). Revisiting the mine-thine problem: A sensitizing exercise for clinic, classroom, and attributional research. *Rehabilitation Psychology, 57*, 113–123.

Dunn, D. S., Fisher, D., & Beard, B. (2013). Disability as diversity rather than (in)difference: Understanding others' experiences through one's own. In D. S. Dunn, R. A. R. Gurung, K. Naufel, & J. H. Wilson (Eds.), *Controversy in the psychology classroom: Using hot topics to foster critical thinking* (pp. 209–223). APA Books.

Dunn, D. S., & Hammer, E. D. (2014). On teaching multicultural psychology. In F. L. Leong, L. Comas-Díaz, G. C. Nagayama Hall, V. C. McLoyd, J. E. Trimble (Eds.), *APA handbook of multicultural psychology: Vol. 1, Theory and research* (pp. 43–58). American Psychological Association. http://doi.org/10.1037/14189-003

Dunn, E., & Norton, M. (2014). *Happy money: The science of happier spending*. Simon & Schuster.

Dunn, D. S., Uswatte, G., & Elliott, T. R. (2009). Happiness, resilience and positive growth following physical disability: Issues for understanding, research, and therapeutic intervention. In S. J. Lopez & C. R. Snyder (Eds.), *Oxford handbook of positive psychology* (2nd ed., pp. 651–664). Oxford University Press.

Dunn, D. S., Uswatte, G., & Elliott, T. R. (2021). Happiness and resilience following physical disability. In C. R. Snyder, S. J. Lopez, L. Edwards, & S. Marques (Eds.), *Oxford handbook of positive psychology* (3rd ed., pp. 928–942). Oxford University Press.

Dunn, D. S., Uswatte, G., Elliott, T. R., Lastres, A., & Beard, B. (2013). A positive psychology of physical disability: Principles and progress. In M. L. Wehmeyer (Ed.), *The Oxford handbook of positive psychology and disability* (pp. 427–441). Oxford University Press.

Dunning, D., Griffin, D. W., Milojkovic, J. D., & Ross, L. (1990). The overconfidence effect in social prediction. *Journal of Personality and Social Psychology, 58*, 568–581.

Eagly, A. H., Ashmore, R. D., Makhijani, M. G., & Longo, L. C. (1991). What is beautiful is good but . . . : A meta-analytic review of research on the physical attractiveness stereotype. *Psychological Bulletin, 110*, 107–128. http://doi.org/10.1037/0033-2909.110.1.109

Eagly, A. H., & Chaiken, S. (1993). *The psychology of attitudes*. Harcourt.

Ehde, D. M. (2010). Application of positive psychology to rehabilitation psychology. In R. G. Frank, M. Rosenthal, & B. Caplan (Eds.), *Handbook of rehabilitation psychology* (pp. 417–424). American Psychological Association. http://doi.org/10.1037/15972-029

Ehde, D. M., Wegener, S. T., Williams, R. M., Ephraim, P. L., Stevenson, J. E., Isenberg, P. J., & MacKenzie, E. J. (2013). Developing, testing, and sustaining rehabilitation interventions via participatory action research. *Archives of Physical Medicine and Rehabilitation, 94*(1), S30–S42. http://doi.org/10.1016/j.apmr.2012.10.025

Eid, M., & Larsen, R. J. (Eds.). (2008). *The science of subjective well-being.* Guilford.

Elliott, T. R., & Kennedy, P. (2004). Treatment of depression following spinal cord injury: An evidence-based review. *Rehabilitation Psychology, 49*, 134–139. http://doi.org/10.1037/0090-5550.49.2.134

Elliott, T. R., & Rath, J. F. (2012). Rehabilitation psychology. In *The Oxford handbook of counseling psychology.* (pp. 679–702). Oxford University Press.

Elliott, T. R., Kurylo, M., & Rivera, P. (2002). Positive growth following acquired physical disability. In C. R. Snyder & S. J. Lopez (Eds.), *Handbook of positive psychology* (pp. 687–699). Oxford University Press.

Emmons, R. A., & McCullough, M. E. (2003). Counting blessings versus burdens: An experimental investigation of gratitude and subjective well-being in daily life. *Journal of Personality and Social Psychology, 84*, 377–389.

Erikson, E. H. (1950). *Childhood and society.* Norton.

Erikson, E. H. (1986). *Identity, youth and crisis.* Norton.

Ernst, F. A. (1987). Contrasting perceptions of distress by research personnel and their spinal cord injured subjects. *American Journal of Physical Medicine, 66*, 12–15.

Festinger, L. A. (1954). A theory of social comparison processes. *Human Relations, 7*, 117–140.

Festinger, L., Pepitone, A., & Newcomb, T. (1952). Some consequences of deindividuation in a group. *Journal of Abnormal and Social Psychology, 47*, 382–389.

Fichten, C. S., Amsel, R., Bourdon, C. V., & Creti, L. (1988). Interaction between college students with various disabilities and their nondisabled peers. *Journal of Applied Rehabilitation Counseling, 19*, 13–20. http://doi.org/10.1037/h0079074

Fichten, C. S., Robillard, K., Tagalakis, V., & Amsel, R. (1991). Casual interaction between college students with various disabilities and their nondisabled peers: The internal dialogue. *Rehabilitation Psychology, 32*, 3–20.

Fine, M., & Asch, A. (1988). Disability beyond stigma: Social interaction, discrimination, and activism. *Journal of Social Issues, 44*, 3–21. http://doi.org/10.1111/j.1540-4560.1988.tb02045.x

Finlay, M., & Lyons, E. (1998). Social identity and people with learning difficulties: Implications for self-advocacy groups. *Disability & Society, 13*(1), 37–51. http://doi.org/10.1080/09687599826902

Fiske, S. T. (2005). Social cognition and the normality of prejudgment. In J. F. Dovidio, P. Glick, & L. A. Rudman (Eds.), *On the nature of prejudice: Fifty years after Allport* (pp. 36–53). Blackwell. http://doi.org/10.1002/9780470773963.ch3

Fiske, S. T. (2011). *Envy up, score down: How status divides us.* Russell Sage Foundation.

Fiske, S. T., Cuddy, A. J. C., Glick, P., & Xu, J. (2002). A model of (often mixed) stereotype content: Competence and warmth respectively follow from perceived status and competition. *Journal of Personality and Social Psychology, 82*, 878–902. http://doi.org/10.1037/0022-3514.82.6.878

Fiske, S. T., & Taylor, S. E. (2014). *Social cognition: From brains to culture* (2nd ed.). Sage. http://doi.org/10.4135/9781446286395

Flaubert, G. (1982). *The letters of Gustave Flaubert, 1857–1880.* (F. Steegmuller, Ed., and Trans.). Harvard University Press.

Fleming, A. R., Roundtree, S. M., & Pierce, K. L. (2024). The evolution of laws and policies in the United States and their impact on disabled people. In I. Marini, A. R. Fleming, & M. Bishop (Eds.), *The psychosocial impact of chronic illness and disability* (8th ed., pp. 85–101). Springer Publishing.

Fleming, A. R., Umucu, E., & Phillips, B. N. (2024). Interventions to improve the well-being of people with disabilities and chronic illness. In I. Marini, A. R. Fleming, & M. Bishop (Eds.), *The psychological and social impact of chronic illness and disability* (8th ed., pp. 401–415). Springer Publishing.

Folkman, S. (Ed.). (2010). *The Oxford handbook of stress, health, and coping*. Oxford University Press.

Forber-Pratt, A., Dunn, D. S., Nario-Redmond, M., Burdick, C. E., & Baeza, M. (in press). Disability identity. In M. Meade, K. Bechtold, & S. Wegener (Eds.), *Oxford handbook of rehabilitation psychology* (2nd ed). Oxford University Press.

Forber-Pratt, A. J., Lyew, D. A., Mueller, C., & Samples, L. B. (2017). Disability identity development: A systematic review of the literature. *Rehabilitation Psychology, 62*(2), 198–210. https://doi.org/10.1037/rep0000134

Forber-Pratt, A. J., Mueller, C. O., & Andrews, E. E. (2018). Disability identity and allyship in rehabilitation psychology: Sit, stand, sign, and show up. *Rehabilitation Psychology, 64*(2), 119–129. https://doi.org/10.1037/rep0000256

Fordyce, W. E. (1971). Behavioral methods in rehabilitation. In W. S. Neff (Ed.), *Rehabilitation psychology*. (pp. 74–108). American Psychological Association. https://doi.org/10.1037/10043-007

Fordyce, W. E. (1976). *Behavioral methods for chronic pain and illness*. Mosby.

Forester, E. M. (1989). *Howards end*. Vintage Books. (Original work published 1910)

Fox, D. D., & Marini, I. (2024). History of treatment toward persons with disabilities in America and abroad. In I. Marini, A. R. Fleming, & M. Bishop (Eds.), *The psychological and social impact of chronic illness and disability* (8th ed.) (pp. 5–16). Springer Publishing.

Frankl, V. E. (1985). *Man's search for meaning* (rev. & updated). Washington Square Press.

Funder, D. (2024). *The personality puzzle* (9th ed.). Norton.

Galanes, P. (2024, February 28). *Social Q's: Why can't my friend accept that my disabled son has a great life?* https://www.nytimes.com/2024/02/28/style/disability-pity-friendship.html

Galatzer-Levy, I. R., Huang, S. H., & Bonanno, G. A. (2018). Trajectories of resilience and dysfunction following potential trauma: A review and statistical evaluation. *Clinical Psychology Review, 63*, 41–55. https://doi.org/10.1016/j.cpr.2018.05.008

Gay, P. (1995). *The enlightenment: The rise of modern paganism*. W. W. Norton.

Gerhart, K. A., Koziel-McLain, J., Lowenstein, S. R., & Whiteneck, G. G. (1994). Quality of life following spinal cord injury: Knowledge and attitudes of emergency care providers. *Annals of Emergency Medicine, 23*, 807–812.

Gernsbacher, M. A. (2017). Editorial perspective: The use of person-first language in scholarly writing may accentuate stigma. *Journal of Child Psychology and Psychiatry, 58*(7), 859–861. https://doi.org/10.1111/jcpp.12706

Gibson, J. (2006). Disability and clinical competency: An introduction. *California Psychologist, 39*, 6–10.

Gilbert, D. T. (1998). Speeding with Ned: A personal view of the correspondence bias. In J. M. Darley & J. Cooper (Eds.), *Attribution and social interaction: The legacy of Edward E. Jones* (pp. 5–66). American Psychological Association. https://doi.org/10.1037/10286-001

Gilbert, D. T., & Malone, P. S. (1995). The correspondence bias. *Psychological Bulletin, 117*(1), 21–38. https://doi.org/10.1037/0033-2909.117.1.21

Gill, C. (1995, Fall). A psychological view of disability culture. *Disability Studies Quarterly, 15* (4), 16–19.

Gill, C. (1997). Four types of integration in disability identity development. *Journal of Vocational Rehabilitation, 9*, 39–46. https://doi.org/0.1016/S1052-2263(97)00020-2

Gill, C., Kewman, D. G., & Brannon, R. W. (2003). Transforming psychological practice and society: Policies that reflect the new paradigm. *American Psychologist, 58*(4), 305–312. https://doi.org/10.1037/0003-066X.58.4.305

Gill, C. J. (1987). A new social perspective on disability and its implications for rehabilitation. *Occupational Therapy in Health Care, 4*(1), 49–55.

Gilovich, T., & Ross, L. (2015). *The wisest one in the room: How you can benefit from social psychology's most powerful insights*. Free Press.

Goffman, E. (1963). *Stigma: Notes on the management of a spoiled identity*. Prentice-Hall.

Goodley, D. (2011). *Disability studies: An interdisciplinary introduction*. Sage.

Gouvier, W. D., Coon, R. C., Todd, M. E., & Fuller, K. H. (1994). Verbal interaction with individuals presenting with or without physical disabilities. *Rehabilitation Psychology, 39*, 263–268. https://doi.org/10.1037/h0080322

Graf, N. M., & Glover, R. L. (2024). Sexuality and disability. In I. Marini, A. R. Fleming, & M. Bishop (Eds.), *The psychological and social impact of chronic illness and disability* (8th ed., pp. 169–195). Springer Publishing.

Groessl, E. J., Kaplan, R. M., Rejeski, W. J., Katula, J. A., Glynn, N. W., King, A. C., Anton, S. D., Walkup, M., Lu, C.-J., Reid, K., Spring, B., & Pahor, M. (2019). Physical activity and performance impact long-term quality of life in older adults at risk for major mobility disability. *American Journal of Preventive Medicine, 56*(1), 141–146. https://doi.org/10.1016/j.amepre.2018.09.006.

Grue, J. (2016). The problem with inspiration porn: A tentative definition and a provisional critique. *Disability & Society, 31*(6), 838–849. https://doi.org/10.1080/09687599.2016.1205473

Gurung, R. A. R, & Neufeld, G. (Eds.). (2022). *Transforming Introductory Psychology: Expert advice on teacher training, course design, and student success*. American Psychological Association.

Hahn, H., & Beaulaurier, R. L. (2001). Attitudes towards disabilities: A research note on activists with disabilities. *Journal of Disability Policy Studies, 12*, 40–46. https://doi.org/10.1177/104420730101200105

Hahn, H., & Belt, T. L. (2004). Disability identity and attitudes towards a cure in a sample of disabled activists. *Journal of Health and Social Behavior, 45*, 453–464. https://doi.org/10.1177/002214650404500407

Hall, K. M., Knudson, S. T., Wright, J., Charlifue, S. W., Graves, D. E., & Warner, P. (1999). Follow-up study of individuals with tetraplegia (C1-C4). 14 to 24 years postinjury. *Archives of Physical Medicine and Rehabilitation, 80*, 1507–1513.

Hamedani, M. G., Markus, H. R., Hetey, R. C., & Eberhardt, J. L. (2024). We built this culture (so we can change it): Seven principles for intentional culture change. *American Psychologist, 79*(3), 384–402. https://doi.org/10.1037/amp0001209

Hamera, E. K., & Shontz, F. C. (1978). Perceived positive and negative effects of life-threatening illness. *Journal of Psychosomatic Research, 22*, 419–424. https://doi.org/10.1016/0022-3999(78)90064-8

Hammell, K. W. (2004). Exploring quality of life following high spinal cord injury: A review and critique. *Spinal Cord, 42*, 491–502. https://doi.org/10.1038/sj.sc.3101636

Hamraie, A. (2017). *Building access: Universal design and the politics of disability*. University of Minnesota Press.

Hanass-Hancock, J., & Alli, F. (2015). Closing the gap: Training for healthcare workers and people with disabilities on the interrelationship of HIV and disability. *Disability and Rehabilitation, 37*(21), 2012–2021.

Hanson, S. L., Bruyere, S., Forber-Pratt, A., Reesman, J., & Sung, C. (2023). Guidelines for assessment and intervention with persons with disabilities: An executive summary. *American Psychologist, 78*(8), 995–1009. https://doi-org/10.1037/amp0001150

Hard, B. M., Dunn, D. S., Hudson, D., Musselman, R., & Richmond, A. (2022). Designing the introductory psychology course: An evidence-informed framework. In R. A. R. Gurung & G. Neufeld (Eds.), *Transforming Introductory Psychology: Expert advice on teacher training, course design, and student success* (pp. 27–56). American Psychological Association.

Heider, F. (1958). *The psychology of interpersonal relations*. Wiley. http://doi.org/10.1037/10628-000

Heinemann, A. W. (1995). Measures of coping and reaction to disability. In L. A. Cushman & M. J. Schhrer (Eds.), *Psychological assessment in medical rehabilitation* (pp. 39–99). American Psychological Association.

Heinrich, J., Heine, S., & Norenzayan, A. (2010). The weirdest people in the world? *Behavioral and Brain Sciences*, *33*, 61–83.

Helson, H. (1964). *Adaptation-level theory*. Harper & Row.

Henderson, G., & Bryan, W. V. (2011). *Psychosocial aspects of disability* (4th ed.). Thomas.

Hendren, S. (2020). *What can a body do? How we meet the built world*. Riverhead Books.

Henrich, J. (2021). *The WEIRDEST people in the world: How the west became psychologically peculiar and particularly prosperous*. Picador.

Hevern, V. W. (2008). Why narrative psychology can't afford to ignore the body. Special Issue: Proceedings of the 2nd Annual Meeting of the Northeastern Evolutionary Psychology Society. *Journal of Social, Evolutionary, and Cultural Psychology*, *2*(4), 217–233.

Hojati, A. (2012). A study of euphemisms in the context of English-speaking media. *International Journal of Linguistics*, *4*, 522–562. http://doi.org/10.5296/ijl.v4i4.2933

Hong, M., & Morgan, A. (2019, February). *An introduction to open science*. Psychological Science Agenda. Retrieved August 18, 2022, from https://www.apa.org/science/about/psa/2019/02/open-science

Hurst, N. P., Jobabputra, P., Hunter, M., Lambert, M., Lochhead, A., & Brown, H. (1994). Validity of Euroqol—a generic health status instrument—in patients with rheumatoid arthritis. *British Journal of Rheumatology*, *33*, 655–662. http://doi.org/10.1093/rheumatology/33.7.655

Iezzoni, L. I., Rao, S. R., Ressalam, J., Bolcic-Jankovic, D., Agaronnik, N. D., Donelan, K., Lagu, T., & Campbell, E. G. (2021). Physicians' perceptions of people with disability and their health care: Study. *Health Affairs*, *40*(2), 297–306. https://doi.org/10.1037/0022-3514.65.3.563

Isen, A. M., & Levin, P. F. (1972). Effects of feeling good on helping: Cookies and kindness. *Journal of Personality and Social Psychology*, *21*, 384–388.

Janoff-Bulman, R. (1992). *Shattered assumptions: Towards a new psychology of trauma*. Free Press.

Jones, E. E., Farina, A., Hastorf, A. H., Markus, H., Miller, D. T., & Scott, R. A. (Eds.). (1984). *Social stigma: The psychology of marked relationships*. Freeman and Company.

Jones, E. E., Kanouse, D. E., Kelley, H. H., Nisbett, R. E., Valins, S., & Weiner, B. (Eds.), (1971). *Attribution: Perceiving the causes of behavior*. General Learning Press.

Jones, E. E., & Nisbett, R. E. (1971). The actor and the observer: Divergent perceptions of the causes of behavior. In E. E. Jones, D. E. Kanouse, H. H. Kelley, R. E. Nisbett, S. Valins, & B. Weiner (Eds), *Attribution: Perceiving the causes of behavior* (pp. 79–94). General Learning Press.

Kahneman, D. (2000). Experienced utility and objective happiness: A moment-based approach. In D. Kahneman & A. Tversky (Eds.), *Choices, values, and frames* (pp. 673–692). Russell Sage Foundation; Cambridge University Press.

Kahneman, D., & Deaton, A. (2010). High income improves evaluation of life but not emotional well-being. *Proceedings of the National Academy of Sciences of the United States of America*, *107*(38), 16489–16493.

Kahneman, D., Diener, E., & Schwartz, N. (Eds.). (1999). *Well-being: The foundations of hedonic psychology*. Russell Sage.

Kahneman, D., & Tversky, A. (1979). Prospect theory: An analysis of decision under risk. *Econometrica*, *47*, 263–291.

Kashdan, T. (2015). What really makes you a happy person? *Psychology Today*. https://www.psychologytoday.com/blog/curious/201508/what-really-makes-you-happy-person

Kasser, T. (2002). *The high price of materialism*. MIT Press.

Keany, K. C., & Glueckauf, R. L. (1993). Disability and value change: An overview and reanalysis of acceptance of loss theory. *Rehabilitation Psychology*, *38*, 199–210. https://doi.org/10.1037/h0080297

Kelley, H. H. (1950). The warm-cold variable in the first impressions of persons. *Journal of Personality*, *18*, 431–439. https://doi.org/10.1111/j.1467-6494.1950.tb01260.x

Kendall, E., & Buys, N. (1998). An integrated model of psychosocial adjustment following acquired disability. *Journal of Rehabilitation*, *64*, 16–20.

Kerr, N. (1961). Understanding the process of adjustment to disability. *Journal of Rehabilitation, 27*(6), 16–18.

Keyes, C. L. M., & Haidt, J. (Eds.). (2003). *Flourishing: Positive psychology and the life well-lived.* American Psychological Association. https://doi.org/10.1037/10594-000

Killingsworth, M. A. (2021). Experienced well-being rises with income, even above $75,000 per year. *Proceedings of the National Academy of Sciences of the United States of America, 118*(4), 1–6. https://doi.org/10.1073/pnas.2016976118

Killingsworth, M. A., Kahneman, D., & Mellers, B. (2023). Income and emotional well-being: A conflict resolved. *Proceedings of the National Academy of Sciences of the United States of America, 120*(10), 1–6. https://doi.org/10.1073/pnas.2208661120

Kitchin, R. (2000). The researched opinions on research: Disabled people and disability research. *Disabilty & Society, 15*(1), 24–47. https://doi.org/10.1080/09687590025757

Kleck, R. F. (1968). Physical stigma and nonverbal cues emitted in face to face interactions. *Human Relations, 21*, 19–28. https://doi.org/10.1177/001872676802100102

Kleve, L., Rumsey, N., Wyn-Williams, M., & White, P. (2002). The effectiveness of cognitive-behavioural interventions provided at Outlook: A disfigurement support unit. *Journal of Evaluation in Clinical Practice, 8*(4), 387–395. https://doi.org/10.1046/j.1365-2753.2002.00348.x

Kohn, N. A., Blumenthal, J. A., & Campbell, A. T. (2013). Supported decision-making: A viable alternative to guardianship. *Dickinson Law Review, 117*, 1111–1157.

Krueger, J. I. (2015). *Happy pie: Intend to become happier and do something about it.* https://www.psychologytoday.com/blog/one-among-many/201503/happy-pie

Kukita, A., Nakamura, J., & Csikszentmihalyi, M. (2022). How experiencing autonomy contributes to a good life. *The Journal of Positive Psychology, 17*(1), 34–45. https://doi.org/10.1080/17439760.2020.1818816

Kurtz, J. L. (2018). Savoring: A positive emotion amplifier. In D. S. Dunn (Ed.), *Positive psychology: Established and emerging issues* (pp. 46–60). Routledge/Taylor & Francis Group. https://doi.org/10.4324/9781315106304-4

Kuzu, D., Ehde, D. M., Waldron-Perrine, B., Whibley, D., & Kratz, A. L. (2024). Exploration of how valued living relates to resilience among people with spinal cord injury. *Rehabilitation Psychology, 69*(2), 94–101. https://doi.org/10.1037/rep0000535

Langer, E. J., & Ngnoumen, C. T. (2018). Mindfulness. In D. S. Dunn (Ed.), *Positive psychology: Established and emerging issues* (pp. 97–111). Routledge.

Larsen, R. J., & Prizmic, Z. (2008). Regulation of emotional well-being: Overcoming the hedonic treadmill. In M. Eid & R. J. Larsen (Ed.), *The science of subjective well-being* (pp. 258–289). Guilford.

Larson, P., & Sachs, P. (2000). A history of division 22. In D. A. Dewsbury (Ed.), *Unification through division: Histories of the divisions of the American Psychological Association* (Vol. 5, pp. 33–58). American Psychological Association.

Lazarus, R. S., & Folkman, S. (1984). *Stress, appraisal, and coping.* Springer.

Leventhal, H., Musumeci, T., & Leventhal, E. (2006). Psychological approaches to the connection of health and behavior. *South African Journal of Psychology, 36*, 666–682.

Leviton, G. (1973). Professional and client viewpoints on rehabilitation issues [Special Issue]. *Rehabilitation Psychology, 20.*

Lewin, K. 1946. Action research and minority problems. *Journal of Social Issues 2*, 34–46. https://doi.org/10.1111/j.1540-4560.1946.tb02295.x

Lewin, K. (1997). *Field theory in social science: Selected theoretical papers* (D. Cartwright, Ed.). American Psychological Association. (Original work published 1951)

Lewin, K. A. (1935). *A dynamic theory of personality.* McGraw-Hill.

Lewin, K. A. (1997). *Resolving social conflicts: Field theory in social science.* American Psychological Association. (Original work published 1948)

Li, L., & Moore, D. (1998). Acceptance of disability and its correlates. *Journal of Social Psychology, 138*(1), 13–25. http://doi.org/10.1080/00224549809600349

Liesener, J. J.m & Mills, J. (1999). An experimental study of disability spread: Talking to an adult in a wheelchair like a child. *Journal of Applied Social Psychology, 29*, 2083–2092. http://doi.org/10.1111/j.1599-1816.1999.tb02296.x

Lindstrom, L., Doren, B., Post, C., & Lombardi, A. (2013). Building career PATHS (postschool achievement through higher skills) for young women with disabilities. *Career Development Quarterly, 61*, 330–338. http://doi.org/10/1002/j.2161-0045.2013.00059.x

Link, B. G., & Phelan, J. C. (2001). Conceptualizing stigma. *Annual Review of Sociology, 27*, 3363–3385. http://doi.org/10.1146/annurev.soc.271.1.363

Linkowski, D. C. (1971). A scale to measure acceptance of disability. *Rehabilitation Counseling Bulletin, 14*, 236–244.

Linville, P. W., & Jones, E. E. (1980). Polarized appraisals of outgroup members. *Journal of Personality and Social Psychology, 52*(4), 663–676. http://doi.org/10.1037/0022-3514.52.4.663

Livneh, H. (1986). A unified approach to existing models of adaptation to disability. I. A model adaptation. *Journal of Applied Rehabilitation Counseling, 17*(1), 5–16, 56.

Livneh, H. (1987). Person-environment congruence: A rehabilitation perspective. *International Journal of Rehabilitation Research, 10*, 3–19. http://doi.org/10.1097/00004356-198703000=00001

Livneh, H., & Antonak, R. F. (1997). *Psychosocial adaptation to chronic illness and disability*. Aspen.

Livneh, H., & Antonak, R. F. (2005). Psychosocial adaptation to chronic illness and disability: A primer for counselors. *Journal of Counseling & Development, 83*(1), 12–20. http://doi.org/10.1002/j.1556-6678.2005.tb00575.x

Livneh, H., Lott, S., & Antonak, R. (2004). Patterns of psychosocial adaptation to chronic illness and disability: A cluster analytic approach. *Psychology, Health, & Medicine, 9*(4), 411–430. http://doi.org/10.1080/13548500420000267030

Locksley, A., Ortiz, V., & Hepburn, C. (1980). Social categorization and discriminatory behavior: Extinguishing the minimal intergroup discrimination effect. *Journal of Personality and Social Psychology, 39* (5), 773–783. doi: 10.1037/0022-3514.39.5.773

Lockwood, P. (2002). Could it happen to you? Predicting the impact of downward comparisons on the self. *Journal of Personality and Social Psychology, 82*(3), 343–358. http://doi.org/10.1037/0022-3514.82.3.343

Lollar, D. J., Horner-Johnson, W., & Froehlich-Grobe, K. (Eds.). (2021). *Public health perspectives on disability: Science, social justice, ethics, and beyond* (2nd ed.). Springer Publishing.

Longmore, P. K. (2003). *Why I burned my book and other essays on disability*. Temple University Press.

Longmore, P. K., & Umansky, L. (Eds.). (2001). *The new disability history: American perspectives*. New York University Press.

Lopez, K. (2021, September 20). *"Crip Camp" co-director James LeBrecht claims CBS and Television Academy deceived him on Emmy ramp*. Indie Wire. https://www.indiewire.com/2021/09/crip-camp-director-deceived-cbs-emmy-ramp-1234666016/?fbclid=IwAR1WcQnTzyu6FZvDgLcFGHa3CZttfW-dEDPSgzVeIVv9hXdtvNcGlCkQQYs

Lucas, R. (2007a). Adaptation and the set-point model of subjective well-being: Does happiness change after major life events? *Current Directions in Psychological Science, 16*, 75–79. http://doi.org/10.1111/j.1467-8721.2007.00479.x

Lucas, R. (2007b). Long-term disability is associated with lasting changes in subjective well-being: Evidence from two nationally representative longitudinal studies. *Journal of Personality and Social Psychology, 92*, 717–730. http://doi.org/10.1037/0022-3514.92.4.717

Lund, E. M. (2021). Even more to handle: Additional sources of stress and trauma for clients from marginalized racial and ethnic groups in the United States during the COVID-19 pandemic. *Counselling Psychology Quarterly, 34*(3–4), 321–330. http://doi.org/10.1080/09515070.2020.1766420

Lund, E. M., Andrews, E. E., & Holt, J. M. (2014). How we treat our own: The experiences and characteristics of psychology trainees with disabilities. *Rehabilitation Psychology, 59*, 367–375.

Lund, E. M., & Ayers, K. B. (2020). Raising awareness of disabled lives and health care rationing during the COVID-19 pandemic. *Psychological Trauma: Theory, Research, Practice, and Policy, 12*(S1), S210–S211. http://doi.org/10.1037/tra0000673

Lund, E. M., Forber-Pratt, A. J., Wilson, C., & Mona, L. R. (2020). The COVID-19 pandemic, stress, and trauma in the disability community: A call to action. *Rehabilitation Psychology, 65*(4), 313–322. https://doi.org/10.1037/rep0000368

Lyubomirsky, S., Dickerhoof, R., Boehm, J. K., & Sheldon, K. M. (2011). Becoming happier takes both a will and a proper way: An experimental longitudinal intervention to boost well-being. *Emotion, 11*(2), 391–402. http://doi.org/10.1037/a0022575

Lyubomirsky, S., & Layous, K. (2013). How do simple positive activities increase well-being? *Current Directions in Psychological Science, 22*(1), 57–62. http://doi.org/10.1177/0963721412469809

Lyubomirsky, S., Sheldon, K. M., & Schkade, D. (2005). Pursuing happiness: The architecture of sustainable change. *Review of General Psychology, 9*, 111–131. http://doi.org/10.1037/1089-2680.9.2.111

Maciver, D., Prior, S., Forsyth, K., Walsh, M., Meiklejohn, A., Irvine, L., & Pentland, D. (2013). Vocational rehabilitation: Facilitating evidence based practice through participatory action research. *Journal of Mental Health, 22*(2), 183–190. http://doi.org/10.3109/09638237.2012.734659

Mackelprang, R. W., & Salsgiver, R. O. (2016). *Disability: A diversity model of approach in human service practice* (3rd ed.). Oxford University Press.

Macrae, C. N., & Bodenhausen, G. V. (2001). Social cognition: Categorical person perception. *British Journal of Social Psychology, 92*, 239–255. http://doi.org/10.1348/000712601162059

Main, C. J., Keefe, F. J., Jensen, M. P., Vlaeyen, J. W. S., & Vowles, K. E. (Eds.). (2015). *Fordyce's behavioral methods for chronic pain and illness: Republished with invited commentaries*. Wolters Kluwer.

Malle, B. F. (2006). The actor-observer asymmetry in attribution: A (surprising) meta-analysis. *Psychological Bulletin, 132*, 895–919. http://doi.org/10.1037/0033-2909.132.6.985

Malle, B. F. (2011). Attribution theories: How people make sense of behavior. In D. Chadee (Ed.), *Theories in social psychology* (pp. 72–95). Wiley-Blackwell.

Manning, R. B. III, Cipollina, R., Lowe, S. R., Bogart, K. R., Ostrove, J. M., Adler, J. M., Nario-Redmond, M. R., & Wang, K. (2023). Barriers to mental health service use among people with disabilities during the COVID-19 pandemic. *Rehabilitation Psychology, 68*(4), 351–361. https://doi.org/10.1037/rep0000512

Marini, I. (1992). The use of humor in counseling as a social skill for clients who are disabled. *Journal of Applied Rehabilitation Counseling, 23*, 30–36.

Marini, I. (2024). Societal attitudes and myths about disability: Improving the social consciousness. In I. Marini, A. R. Fleming, & M. Bishop (Eds.), *The psychological and social impact of chronic illness and disability* (8th ed., pp. 17–35). Springer Publishing.

Marini, I., & Villarreal, L. A. (2024). Theories of adjustment and adaptation to disability. In I. Marini, A. R. Fleming, & M. Bishop (Eds.), *The psychological and social impact of chronic illness and disability* (8th ed., pp. 123–146). Springer Publishing.

Marks, D. (1999). *Disability: Controversial debates and psychosocial perspectives*. Routledge.

Marrow, A. J. (1977). *The practical theorist: The life and work of Kurt Lewin*. Teachers College Press.

Maruyama, G., & Van Boekel, M. (2014). Action research. In D. S Dunn (Ed.), *Oxford bibliographies: Psychology*. https://doi.org/10.1093/OBO/9780199828340-0149

Mason, L., & Muhlenkamp, A. (1976). Patients' self-reported affective states following loss and caregivers' expectations of patients' affective states. *Rehabilitation Psychology, 23*, 72–76. https://doi.org/10.1037/h0090904

Masten, A. S., Cutuili, J. J., Herbers, J. E., & Reed, M.-G. J. (2009). Resilience in development. In S. J. Lopez & C. R. Snyder (Ed.), *Oxford handbook of positive psychology* (2nd ed., pp. 171–131). Oxford University Press.

McBryde Johnson, H. (2003, February 16). Unspeakable conversations. *The New York Times Magazine, 152*, 74–79.

McBryde Johnson, H. (2005). *Too late to die young: Nearly true tales from a life*. Henry Holt.

McColl, M. A., Forster, D., Shortt, S. E., Hunter, D., Dorland, J., Godwin, M. & Rosser, W. (2008). Physician experiences providing primary care to people with disabilities. *Healthcare Policy, 4*(1), e129–e147. https://doi.org/10.12927/hcpol.2008.19989

McDonald, K. E., & Raymaker, D. M. (2013). Paradigm shifts in disability and health: Toward more ethical public health research. *American Journal of Public Health, 103*(12), 2165–2173. https://doi.org/10.2105/ajph.2013.301286

McGinnis, J. M., & Foege, W. H. (1993). Actual causes of death in the United States. *Journal of the American Medical Association, 270*, 2207–2212. http://doi.org/10.1001/jama.1993.03510180077038

Meade, M., Becthold, K., & Wegener, S. (Eds.) (in press). *Oxford handbook of rehabilitation psychology*. Oxford University Press.

Mesman, E., Vreeker, A., & Hillegers, M. (2021). Resilience and mental health in children and adolescents: an update of the recent literature and future directions. *Current Opinion in Psychiatry, 34*(6), 586–592. https://doi.org/10.1097/YCO.0000000000000741

Miles, J. R., & Fassinger, R. E. (2021). Creating a public psychology through a scientist-practitioner-advocacy training model. *American Psychologist, 76*(8), 1232–1247. https://doi.org/10.1037/amp0000855

Miller, G. A. (1969). Psychology as a means of promoting human welfare. *American Psychologist, 24*(12), 1063–1075. https://doi.org/10.1037/h0028988

Miller, G. A. (1970). "Presidential addresses of Miller and Walker": Reply. *American Psychologist, 25*(5), 470–471. https://doi.org/10.1037/h0037747

Millington, M. J. (2012). Basic do's and don'ts in counseling persons with disabilities. In I. Marini, N. M. Glover-Graf, & M. J. Millington (Eds.), *Psychosocial aspects of disability: Insider perspectives and counseling strategies* (pp. 465–480). Springer.

Moore, G. E. (1971). *Principia ethica*. Cambridge University Press. (Original work published 1903).

Myers, W. A. (1970). Comment: Presidential addresses of Miller and Walker [Special Issue: The Place of Psychology in the Universe]. *American Psychologist, 25*(5), 469–470.

Nakamura, J., & Csikszentmihalyi, M. (2002). The concept of flow. In C. R. Snyder & S. J. Lopez (Eds.), *Handbook of positive psychology* (pp. 89–105). Oxford.

Nario-Redmond, M. R. (2020). *Ableism: The causes and consequences of disability prejudice*. Wiley-Blackwell.

Nario-Redmond, M. R., Noel, J. G, & Fern, E. (2013). Redefining disability, reimagining the self: Disability identification predicts self-esteem and strategic responses to stigma. *Self and Identity, 12*(5), 468–488. https://doi.org/10.1080/15298868.2012.681118

Nario-Redmond, M. R. & Oleson, K. C. (2016). Disability group identification, disability-rights advocacy: Contingencies among emerging and other adults. *Emerging Adulthood, 4*(3), 207–218. https://doi.org/10.1177/2167696815579830

National Council on Disability. (2007). *The impact of the Americans with Disabilities Act: Assessing the progress toward achieving the goals of the Americans with Disabilities Act*. Retrieved from http://www.ncd.gov/publications/2007/07262007

Ne'eman, A. (2020, March 23). Disabled in the coronavirus crisis: "I will not apologize for my needs." *New York Times*. https://www.nytimes.com/2020/03/23/opinion/coronavirus-ventilators-triage-disability.html

Nelson, R. G. (2022). *How a virus exposed the myth of rugged individualism*. Scientific American.

Nelson, G., Ochocka, J., Griffin, K., & Lord, J. (1998). "Nothing about me, without me": Participatory action research with self-help/mutual aid organizations for psychiatric consumer/survivors. *American Journal of Community Psychology, 26*(6), 881–912. https://doi.org/10.1023/a:1022298129812

Nelson, S. K., Kushlev, K., English, T., Dunn, E. W., & Lyubomirsky, S. (2013). In defense of parenthood: Children are associated with more joy than misery. *Psychological Science, 24*(1), 3–10. https://doi.org/10.1177/0956797612447798

Nestle, J., Howell, C., & Wilchins, R. A. (Eds.). (2002). *Gender-Queer: Voices from beyond the sexual binary*. Alyson Books.

Neville, H. A., Ruedas-Gracia, N., Lee, B. A., Ogunfemi, N., Maghsoodi, A. H., Mosley, D. V., LaFromboise, T. D., & Fine, M. (2021). The public psychology for liberation training model: A call to transform the discipline. *American Psychologist, 76*(8), 1248–1265. https://doi.org/10.1037/amp0000887

Newman, M., & LaBrecht, J. (codirectors). (2020). *Crip camp* [Film]. Higher Ground.

New York Times. (2024, February 4). Witness: Portraits of the people living in the news, p. C2.

Nielsen, D. (2013). Universal design in first-year composition: Why do we need it, how can we do it? *The CEA Forum, 42*, 3–29.

Niemiec, R. M. (2013). VIA character strengths: research and practice (the first 10 years). In H. Knoop & A. Fave (Eds.), *Well-being and cultures: Perspectives from positive psychology* (pp. 11–29). Springer Science + Business Media. https://doi.org/10.1007/978-94-007-4611-4_2

Nierenberg, B., Mayersohn, G., Serpa, S., Holovatyk, A., Smith, E., & Cooper, S. (2016). Application of well-being therapy to people with disability and chronic illness. *Rehabilitation Psychology, 61*(1), 32–43. https://doi.org/10.1037/rep0000060

Nisbett, R. E. (1980). The trait construct in lay and professional psychology. In L. Festinger (Ed.), *Retrospections on social psychology* (pp. 109–130). Oxford University Press.

Nisbett, R. E., & Ross, L. (1980). *Human inference: Strategies and shortcomings of social judgment*. Prentice-Hall.

Nisbett, R. E., & Valins, S. (1972). Perceiving the causes of one's own behavior. In E. E. Jones, D. E. Kanouse, H. H. Kelley, R. E. Nisbett, S. Valins, & B. Weiner (Eds.), *Attribution: Perceiving the causes of behavior* (pp. 63–78). General Learning Press.

Nisbett, R. E., & Wilson, T. D. (1977). Telling more than we can know: Verbal reports on mental processes. *Psychological Review, 84*, 231–259. https://doi.org/10.1037/0033-295X.84.3.231

Norman, D. (2013). *The design of everyday things* (revised and expanded ed.). Basic Books.

Oakes, P. (2001). The root of all evil in intergroup relations? Unearthing the categorization process. In R. Brown & S. L. Gaertner (Eds.), *Blackwell handbook of social psychology: Intergroup processes* (pp. 3–21). Blackwell.

O'Brien, E., Kristal, A. C., Ellsworth, P. C., & Schwarz, N. (2018). (Mis)imagining the good life and the bad life: Envy and pity as a function of the focusing illusion. *Journal of Experimental Social Psychology, 75*, 41–53. https://doi.org/10.1016/j.jesp.2017.10.002

Olkin, R. (1999). *What psychotherapists should know about disability*. Guilford Press.

Olkin, R. (2002). Could you hold the door for me? Including disability in diversity. *Cultural Diversity and Ethnic Minority Psychology, 8*(2), 130–137. https://doi.org/10.1037/1099-9809.8.2.130

Olkin, R. (2007). Disability-affirmative therapy and case formulation: A template for understanding disability in a clinical context (case study). *Counseling and Human Development*. https://www.highbeam.com/doc/1G1-175350872.html

Olkin, R. (2017). *Disability-affirmative therapy*. Oxford University Press.

Olkin, R., & Pledger, C. (2003). Can disability studies and psychology join hands? *American Psychologist, 58*(4), 296–304. https://doi.org/10.1037/0003-066X.58.4.296

Oyserman, D., Elmore, K., & Smith, G. (2012). Self, self-concept, and identity. In M. R. Leary & J. P. Tangney (Eds.), *Handbook of self and identity* (2nd ed., pp. 69–104). Guilford.

Paluck, E. L., Green, S. A., & Green, D. P. (2019). The contact hypothesis re-evaluated. *Behavioural Public Policy, 3*(2), 129–158. https://doi.org/10.1017/bpp.2018.25

Peacock, G. (2019). *Addressing gaps in health care for individuals with intellectual disabilities (Event ID: 4168516)*. CDC Public Health Grand Rounds, Centers for Disease Control and Prevention. https://www.cdc.gov/grand-rounds/pp/2019/20191015-intellectual-disabilities-H.pdf

Peña-Guzmán, D. M., & Reynolds, J. M. (2019). The harm of ableism: Medical error and epistemic injustice. *Kennedy Institute of Ethics Journal, 29*(3), 204–242. https://doi.org/10.1353/ken.2019.0023

Pennebaker, J. W. (1997). *Opening up: The healing power of expressing emotions* (rev. ed.). Guilford.

Pennebaker, J. W. (2004). *Writing to heal: A guided journal for recovering from trauma & emotional upheaval.* New Harbinger Publications.

Perrin, P. B., Goldberg, L. D., & Pierce, B. S. (2019). Multicultural issues and international perspectives on disability. In L. A., Brenner, S. A. Reid-Arndt, T. R. Elliott, R. G Frank, & B. Caplan (Eds.), *Handbook of rehabilitation psychology* (3rd ed., pp. 157–169). American Psychological Association.

Peterson, C. (2013). *Pursuing the good life: 100 reflections on positive psychology.* Oxford University Press.

Peterson, D. B., & Rosenthal, D. R. (2005). The International Classification of Functioning, Disability, and Health (ICF) as an allegory for history and systems in rehabilitation education. *Rehabilitation Education, 19,* 75–80.

Peterson, C., & Park, N. (2011). Character strengths and virtues: Their role in well-being. In S. I. Donalson, M. Csikszentmihalyi, & J. Nakamura (Eds.), *Applied positive psychology: Improving everyday life, health, schools, work, and society* (pp. 49–62). Routledge/Taylor & Francis Group.

Peterson, C., & Park, N. (2012). Character strengths and the life of meaning. In P. P. Wong (Ed.), *The human quest for meaning: Theories, research, and applications* (2nd ed., pp. 277–295). Routledge/Taylor & Francis Group.

Peterson, C., & Seligman, M. E. P. (2004). *Character strengths and virtues: A handbook and classification.* American Psychological Association.

Pettigrew, T. F., & Tropp, L. R. (2006). A meta-analytic test of intergroup contact theory. *Journal of Personality and Social Psychology, 90*(5), 751–783. https://doi.org/10.1037/0022-3514.90.5.751

Pettigrew, T. F., Tropp, L. R., Wagner, U., & Christ, O. (2011). Recent advances in intergroup contact theory. *International Journal of Intercultural Relations, 35*(3), 271–280. https://doi.org/10.1016/j.ijintrel.2011.03.001

Pfeiffer, B. B. (1991). *Frank Lloyd Wright.* Taschen Books.

Pfeiffer, B. B. (2009). *Frank Lloyd Wright 1943–1959: The complete works.* Taschen.

Pierce, C. M., Carew, J. V., Pierce-Gonzalez, D., & Will, D. (1977). An experiment in racism: TV commercials. *Education and Urban Society, 10*(1), 61–87.

Postmes, T., & Spears, R. (1998). Deindividuation and antinormative behavior: A meta-analysis. *Psychological Bulletin, 123,* 238–259. https://doi.org/10.1037/0033-2909.123.3.238

Powell, J. J. W. (2013). From ableism to accessibility in the universal design university. *Review of Disability Studies: An International Journal, 8*(4), 29–41.

Pronin, E., Gilovitch, T., & Ross, L. (2004). Objectivity in the eye of the beholder: Divergent perceptions of bias in self versus others. *Psychological Review, 111*(3), 781–799. https://doi.org/10.1037/0033-295X.111.3.781

Pronin, E., Lin, D. Y., & Ross, L. (2002). The bias blind spot: Perceptions of bias in self versus others. *Personality and Social Psychology Bulletin, 28*(3), 369–381.

Pruett, S. R., & Chan, F. (2006). The development and psychometric validation of the Disability Attitudes Implicit Association Test. *Rehabilitation Psychology, 51,* 202–213.

Putnam, M. (2005). Conceptualizing disability: Developing a framework for political disability identity. *Journal of Disability Policy Studies, 16*(3), 188–198. https://doi.org/10.1177/10442073050160030601

Putnam, R. D. (2001). *Bowling alone: The collapse and revival of American community.* Simon & Schuster.

Quale, A. J., & Schanke, A.-K. (2010). Resilience in the face of coping with a severe physical injury: A study of trajectories of adjustment in a rehabilitation setting. *Rehabilitation Psychology, 55,* 12–22. https://doi.org/10.1037/a0018415

Raskind, M. H., Margalit, M., & Higgins, E. L. (2006). "My LD": Children's voices on the internet. *Learning Disability Quarterly*, *29*(4), 253–268.

Rath, J. F., & Elliott, T. R. (2011). Psychological models in rehabilitation psychology. In P. Kennedy (Ed.), *The Oxford handbook of rehabilitation psychology* (pp. 32–46). Oxford University Press.

Rath, J. R., Dunn, D. S., & Elliott, T. R. (in press). Psychological models in rehabilitation psychology. In M. Meade, K. Becthold, & S. Wegener (Eds.), *Oxford Handbook of Rehabilitation Psychology*. Oxford University Press.

Ravesloot, C., Seekins, T., Traci, M., Boehm, T., White, G., Witten, M. H., Mayer M., & Monson, J. (2016). Living well with a disability, a self-management program. *Morbidity and Mortality Weekly Report/Supplements*, *65*(1), 61–67. http://doi.org/10.15585/mmwr.su6501a10.

Richmond, A. R., Boysen, G. A., Hudson, D. L., Gurung, R. A. R., Naufel, K. Z., Neufeld, G., Landrum, R. E., Dunn, D. S., & Beers, M. (2021). The introductory psychology census: A national study. *Scholarship of Teaching and Learning in Psychology*, *7*(3), 163–180.

Riessman, C. K. (2008). *Narrative methods for the human sciences*. Sage.

Riis, J., Lowenstein, G., Baron, J., Jepson, C., Fagerlin, A., & Ubel, P. A. (2005). Ignorance of hedonic adaptation to hemodialysis: A study using ecological momentary assessment. *Journal of Experimental Psychology: General*, *134*, 3–9. http://doi.org/10.1037/0096-3445.134.1.3

Robey, K., Beckley, L., & Kirschner, M. (2006). Implicit infantilizing attitudes about disability. *Journal of Developmental and Physical Disabilities*, *18*, 441–453.

Roessler, R., & Bolton, B. (1978). *Psychosocial adjustment to disability*. University Park Press.

Ross, L. (1977). The intuitive psychologist and his shortcomings: Distortions in the attribution process. In L. Berkowitz (Ed.), *Advances in experimental social psychology* (vol. 10, pp. 174–221). Academic Press. http://doi.org/10.1016/S0065-2601(08)60357-3

Ross, L. (2018). From the fundamental attribution error to the truly fundamental attribution error and beyond: My research journey. *Perspectives on Psychological Science*, *13*(6), 750–769. http://doi.org/10.1177/1745691618769855

Ross, L., Greene, D., & House, P. (1977). The false consensus effect: An egocentric bias in social perception and attribution processes. *Journal of Experimental Social Psychology*, *13*, 279–301.

Ross, L., & Nisbett, R. E. (1991). *The person in the situation*. McGraw-Hill.

Ross, L., & Ward, A. (1996). Naive realism in everyday life: Implications for social conflict and misunderstanding. In T. Brown, E. S. Reed & E. Turiel (Eds.), *Values and Knowledge* (pp. 103–135). Erlbaum.

Rusalem, H. (1976). A personalized recent history of vocational rehabilitation in America. In H. Rusalem & D. Malikin (Eds.), *Contemporary vocational rehabilitation* (pp. 29–45). New York University Press.

Ryan, R. M., & Deci, E. L. (2001). On happiness and human potentials: A review of research on hedonic and eudaimonic well-being. *Annual Review of Psychology*, *52*, 141–166.

Ryff, C. D. (1989). Happiness is everything, or is it? Explorations on the meaning of psychological well-being. *Journal of Personality and Social Psychology*, *57*, 1069–1081.

Ryff, C. D., & Singer, B. H. (2008). Know thyself and become what you are: A eudaimonic approach to psychological well-being. *Journal of Happiness Studies*, *9*, 13–39.

Sackett, D. L., & Torrance, G. W. (1978). The utility of different health states as perceived by the general public. *Journal of Chronic Diseases*, *31*, 697–704. http://doi.org/10.1016/0021-9681(78)90072-3

Saluny, S. (2011, February 10). In a multicultural nation, many ways to tally. *New York Times*, pp. A1, A17.

Schulz, R., & Decker, S. (1985). Long-term adjustment to physical disability: The role of social support, perceived control, and self-blame. *Journal of Personality and Social Psychology*, *48*, 1162–1172. http://doi.org/10.1037/0022-3514.48.5.1162

Scotch, R. (2002). Paradigms of American social research on disability: What's new? *Disability Studies Quartertly*, *22*(2), 23–34. http://doi.org/10.18061/dsq.v22i2.342

Seligman, M. E. P. (2002). *Authentic happiness: Using the new positive psychology to realize your potential for lasting fulfillment*. Free Press.

Seligman, M. E. P., & Czsikszentmihalyi, M. (2000). Positive psychology: An introduction. *American Psychologist, 55*, 5–14. http://doi.org/10.1037/0003-066X.55.1.5

Serlin, D. (2015). Constructing autonomy: Smart homes for disabled veterans and the politics of normative citizenship. *Critical Military Studies, 1*(1), 38–46. http://doi.org/10.1080/23337486.2015.1005392

Shapiro, J. P. (1994). *No pity: People with disabilities forging a new civil rights movement*. Broadway Books.

Shavelson, R. J., Hubner, J. J., & Stanton, G. C. (1976). Self-concept: Validation of construct interpretations. *Review of Educational Research, 46*, 407–411.

Sheldon, K. M. (2018). Understanding the good life: Eudaimonic living involves well-doing, not well-being. In J. Forgas & R. Baumeister (Eds.), *Sydney symposium 2017: The social psychology of the good life*. Psychology Press.

Sheldon, K. M., & Lyubomirsky, S. (2012). The challenge of staying happier: Testing the hedonic adaptation prevention model. *Personality and Social Psychology Bulletin, 38*(5), 670–680. http://doi.org/0.1177/0146167212436400

Sheldon, K. M., & Lyubomirsky, S. (2021). Revisiting the Sustainable Happiness Model and Pie Chart: Can happiness be successfully pursued? *The Journal of Positive Psychology, 16*(2), 145–154. http://doi.org/10.1080/17439760.2019.1689421

Shontz, F. (1982). Adaptation to chronic illness and disability. In T. Millon, C. Green, & R. Meagher (Eds.), *Handbook of clinical health psychology* (pp.153–172). Plenum Press. http://doi.org/10.1007/978-1-4613-3412-5_8

Shontz, F. C. (1977). Six principles relating disability and psychological adjustment. *Rehabilitation Psychology, 24*(4), 207–210. https://doi.org/10.1037/h0090933

Shontz, F. C., & Wright, B. A. (1980). The distinctiveness of rehabilitation psychology. *Professional Psychology, 11*(6), 919–924. https://doi.org/10.1037/0735-7028.11.6.919

Siebers, T. (2011). *Disability theory*. University of Michigan Press.

Simon, H. A. (1969). *The sciences of the artificial* (3rd ed.). MIT Press.

Smedema, S., Bakken-Gillen, S. K., & Dalton, J. (2009). Psychosocial adaptation to chronic illness and disability: Models and measurement. In F. Chan, E. Da Silva Cardoso, & J. A. Chronister (Eds.), *Understanding psychosocial adjustment to chronic illness and disability: A handbook for evidence-based practitioners in rehabilitation* (pp. 51–73). Springer.

Smith, D. M., Loewenstein, G., Jankovic, A., & Ubel, P. A. (2009). Happily hopeless: Adaptation to a permanent, but not a temporary, disability. *Health Psychology, 28*, 787–791. http://doi.org/10.1037/a0016624

Snyder, C. R., & Lopez, S. J. (Eds.). (2002). *Handbook of positive psychology*. Oxford University Press.

Snyder, C. R., Lopez, S. J., Edwards, L., & Marques, S. (Eds.). (2021). *Oxford handbook of positive psychology* (3rd ed.). Oxford University Press.

Snyder, M., Tanke, E. D., & Berscheid, E. (1977). Social perception and interpersonal behavior: On the self-fulfilling nature of stereotypes. *Journal of Personality and Social Psychology, 35*, 656–666. http://doi.org/10.1037/022-3514.35.9.656

Stapel, D. A., & Kooman, W. (2000). How far do we go beyond the information given? The impact of knowledge activation on interpretation and inference. *Journal of Personality and Social Psychology, 78*, 19–37. http://doi.org/10.1037/0022-3514.78.1.19

Statista. (2024, January 10). *Disability in the U.S.: statistics and facts*. https://www.statista.com/topics/4380/disability-in-the-us/#topicOverview

Steele, C. M. (1997). A threat in the air: How stereotypes shape intellectual identity and performance. *American Psychologist, 52*, 613–629. http://doi.org/10.1037/0003-066X.52.6.613

Steele, C. M. (2011). *Whistling Vivaldi: How stereotypes affect us and what we can do*. Norton.

Steinfeld, E., & Maisel, J. L. (2012). *Universal design: Creating inclusive environments*. John Wiley & Sons.

Stiers, W. (2016). Teaching the foundational principles of rehabilitation psychology. *Rehabilitation Psychology, 61*(1), 54–64. http://doi.org/10.1037/rep0000078

Stiers, W. (2019). Education and training. In L. A. Brenner, S. A. Reid-Arndt, T. R. Elliott, R. G. Frank, & B. Caplan (Eds.), *Handbook of rehabilitation psychology* (3rd ed.). American Psychological Association.

Stodden, R. A., Stodden, N. J., Kim-Rupnow, W. S., Thai, N. D., & Galloway, L. M. (2003). Providing effective support services for culturally and linguistically diverse persons with disabilities: Challenges and recommendations. *Journal of Vocational Rehabilitation, 18*(3), 177–189.

Story, M., Mueller, J., & Mace, R. (1998). The universal design file: Designing for people of all ages and abilities. North Carolina State University Center for Universal Design. https://files.eric.ed.gov/fulltext/ED460554.pdf

Sue, D. W., Alsaidi, S., Awad, M. N., Glaeser, E., Calle, C. Z., & Mendez, N. (2019). Disarming racial microaggressions: Microintervention strategies for targets, White allies, and bystanders. *American Psychologist, 74*(1), 128–142. http://doi.org/10.1037/amp0000296

Sue, D. W., Calle, C. Z., Mendez, N., Alsaidi, S., & Glaeser, E. (2021). *Microintervention strategies: What you can do to disarm and dismantle individual and systemic racism and bias*. J. W. Wiley.

Sue, D. W., Capodilupo, C. M., Torino, G. C., Bucceri, J. M., Holder, A. M. B., Nadal, K. L., & Esquilin, M. (2007). Racial microaggressions in everyday life: Implications for clinical practice. *American Psychologist, 62*(4), 271–286. https://doi.org/10.1037/0003-066X.62.4.271

Sue, D. W., & Spanierman, L. B. (2020). *Microaggressions in everyday life*, 2nd ed. John Wiley & Sons.

Syed, M. (2021, June 10). *WEIRD times: Three reasons to stop using a silly acronym.* Get Syeducated. Retrieved September 6, 2024, from https://getsyeducated.blogspot.com/2024/09/weird-times-three-reasons-to-stop-using.html

Tackett, M. J., Nash, L., Stucky, K. J., & Nierenberg, B. (2016). Supervision in rehabilitation psychology: Application of Beatrice Wright's value-laden beliefs and principles. *Rehabilitation Psychology, 61*(1), 74–81. http://doi.org/10.1037/rep0000070

Tait, R., & Silver, R. C. (1989). Coming to terms with major negative events. In J. S. Uleman & J. A. Bargh (Eds.), *Unintended thought* (pp. 351–382). Guilford.

Tajfel, H. (2001). Experiments in intergroup discrimination. In M. A. Hogg & D. Abrams (Eds.), *Intergroup relations: Essential readings*. (pp. 178–187). Psychology Press.

Tajfel, H., Billig, M. G., Bundy, R. P., & Flament, C. (1971). Social categorization and intergroup behavior. *European Journal of Social Psychology, 1* (2), 149–178. doi: 10.1002/ejsp.2420010202

Tate, D. G., & Pledger, C. (2003). An integrative conceptual framework of disability: New directions for research. *American Psychologist, 58*(4), 919–924. http://doi.org/10.1037/0003-066X.58.4.289

Taylor, S. E., Kemeny, M. E., Reed, G. M., Bower, J. E., & Gruenewald, T. L. (2000). Psychological resources, positive illusions, and health. *American Psychologist, 55*, 99–109.

Taylor, S. E., Lichtman, R. R., & Wood, J. V. (1984). Attributions, beliefs about control, and adjustment to breast cancer. *Journal of Personality and Social Psychology, 46*, 489–502. http://doi.org/10.1037/0022-3514.46.3.489

Taylor, S. E., & Lobel, M. (1989). Social comparison activity under threat: Downward evaluation and upward contacts. *Psychological Review, 96*(4), 569–575. http://doi.org/10.1037/0033-295X.96.4.569

TED. (2016, August). *Elsie Roy: When we design for disability, we all benefit* [Video]. YouTube. https://www.youtube.com/watch?v=g2m97gPI7oI

Tennen, H., & Affleck, G. (2002). Benefit-finding and benefit-reminding. In C. R. Snyder & S. J. Lopez (Eds.), *Handbook of positive psychology* (pp. 584–597). Oxford University Press.

Terrill, A. L., Mackenzie, J., Einerson, J., & Reblin, M. (2019). Resilience and disability: Intrapersonal, interpersonal, and social environment factors. In D. S. Dunn (Ed.), *Understanding the experience of disability: Perspectives from social and rehabilitation psychology* (pp. 313–327). Oxford University Press.

Thayer, R. E. (2001). *Calm energy: How people regulate mood with food and exercise.* Oxford University Press.

Thompson, S. C., & Janigian, A. S. (1988). Life schemes: A framework for understanding the search for meaning. *Journal of Social and Clinical Psychology, 7*, 260–280. http://doi.org/10.1521/jscp.1988.7.2-3.260

Torre, M. E., Fine, M., Stoudt, B. G., & Fox, M. (2012). Critical participatory action research as public science. In H. Cooper, P. M. Camic, D. L. Long, A. T. Panter, D. Rindskopf, & K. J. Sher (Eds.), *APA handbook of research methods in psychology, Vol 2. Research designs: Quantitative, qualitative, neuropsychological, and biological* (pp. 171–184). American Psychological Association.

Trieschmann, R. B. (1988). *Spinal cord injuries: Psychological, social, and vocational rehabilitation* (2nd ed.). Demos.

Trost, Z., Sturgeon, J. A., Azuero, C., Monden, K., & Scott, W. (2019). Perceived injustice and disability. In D. S. Dunn (Ed.), *Understanding the experience of disability: Perspectives from social and rehabilitation psychology* (pp. 331–346). Oxford University Press.

Tsang, H. H., Chan, F., & Chan, C. H. (2004). Factors influencing occupational therapy students' attitudes toward persons with disabilities: A conjoint analysis. *American Journal of Occupational Therapy, 58*(4), 426–434. http://doi.org/10.5014/ajot.58.4.426

Tugade, M. M., & Fredrickson, B. L. (2004). Resilient individuals use positive emotions to bounce back from negative emotional experiences. *Journal of Personality and Social Psychology, 86*, 320–333.

Twain, M. (1899). *Christian Science and the book of Mrs. Eddy.* https://americanliterature.com/author/mark-twain/short-story/christian-science-and-the-book-of-mrs-eddy

Ubel, P. A., Lowenstein, G., & Jepson, C. (2003). Whose quality of life? A commentary exploring discrepancies between health state evaluations and the general public. *Quality of Life Research, 27*, 599–607. http://doi.org/10.1023/A:1025119931010

Vaillant, G. E. (1995). *Adaptation to life.* Harvard University Press.

Vallone, R., Griffin, D., Lin, S., & Ross, L. (1990). Overconfident prediction of future actions and outcomes by self and others. *Journal of Personality and Social Psychology, 58*, 582–592.

Van Boven, L., & Ashworth, L. (2007). Looking forward, looking back: Anticipation is more evocative than retrospection. *Journal of Experimental Psychology: General, 136*, 289–300.

Vash, C. L. (1981). *The psychology of disability.* Springer.

Vash, C. L., & Crewe, N. M. (2004). *Psychology of disability* (2nd ed.). Springer.

Walton, G. M., & Wilson, T. D. (2018). Wise interventions: Psychological remedies for social and personal problems. *Psychological Review, 125*(5), 617–655. http://doi.org/10.1037/rev0000115

Wanberg, C. R. (2012). The individual experience of unemployment. *Annual Review of Psychology, 63*, 369–396. http://doi.org/10.1146/annurev-psych-120710-100500

Wang, K., Manning, R. B. III, Bogart, K. R., Adler, J. M., Nario-Redmond, M. R., Ostrove, J. M., & Lowe, S. R. (2022). Predicting depression and anxiety among adults with disability during the COVID-19 pandemic. *Rehabilitation Psychology, 67*, 179–188. https://doi.org/10.1037/rep0000434

Wang, P. P., Badley, E. M., & Gignac, M. (2006). Exploring the role of contextual factors in disability models. *Disability and Rehabilitation, 28*(2), 135–140. https://doi.org/10.1080/09638280500167761

Waterman, A. S. (1993). Two conceptions of happiness: Contrasts of personal expressiveness (eudaemonia) and hedonic enjoyment. *Journal of Personality and Social Psychology, 64*, 678–691.

Weeber, J. E. (2004). *Disability community leaders' disability identity development: A journey of integration and expansion* (Unpublished doctoral dissertation). North Carolina State University, Raleigh.

Wegner, D. M., & Gilbert, D. T. (2000). Social psychology: The science of human experience. In H. Bless & J. P. Forgas (Eds.), *The message within: The role of subjective experience in social cognition and behavior* (pp. 1–9). Psychology Press.

Wehmeyer, M. L. (Ed.). (2013). *Oxford handbook of positive psychology and disability*. Oxford University Press.

Wehmeyer, M. L. (2019). A social psychology of self-determination and disability. In D. S. Dunn (Ed.), *Understanding the experience of disability: Perspectives from social and rehabilitation psychology* (pp. 300–312). Oxford University Press.

Wehmeyer, M. L., & Dunn, D. S. (2022a). Introduction and overview of the International Classification of Functioning, Disability, and Health. In M. L. Wehmeyer & D. S. Dunn (Eds.), *The positive psychology of personal factors: Implications for understanding disability* (pp. 1–14). Lexington Books/Rowman & Littlefield.

Wehmeyer, M. L., & Dunn, D. S. (Eds.). (2022b). *The positive psychology of personal factors: Implications for understanding disability*. Lexington Books/Rowman & Littlefield.

Wehmeyer, M. L., & Dunn, D. S. (in press). Conceptualizing disability: Positive psychology and the ICF Model. In E. E. Andrews, K. Ayers, D. S. Dunn, & M. L. Wehmeyer (Eds.), *Oxford handbook of positive psychology and disability* (2nd ed.). Oxford University Press.

Weiten, W., Dunn, D. S., & Hammer, E. Y. (2024). *Psychology applied to modern life: Adjustment in the 21st century* (13th ed.). Cengage.

West, J. (2023). *Advocating for the common good: People, politics, process, and policy on Capitol Hill*. Rowman & Littlefield.

White, C. A., Uttl, B., & Holder, M. D. (2019). Meta-analyses of positive psychology interventions: The effects are much smaller than previously reported. *PLoS ONE, 14*(5), e0216588.

White, R. K., Wright, B. A., & Dembo, T. (1948). Studies in adjustment to visible injuries: Evaluation of curiosity by the injured. *Journal of Abnormal and Social Psychology, 43*, 13–28. https://doi.org/10.1037/h0057775

Whiteman, M., & Lukoff, I. F. (1965). Attitudes toward blindness and other physical handicaps. *Journal of Social Psychology, 66*, 133–145. https://doi.org/10.1080/00224545.1965.9919629

Wilder, D. A. (1986). Social categorization: Implications for creation and reduction of intergroup bias. In L. Berkowitz (Ed.), *Advances in experimental social psychology* (Vol. 19, pp. 291–355). Academic Press.

Wiley, S., Philogène, G., & Revenson, T. A. (Eds.). (2012). *Social categories in everyday experience*. American Psychological Association. https://doi.org/10.1037/13488-000

Williamson, G. M. (1998). The central role of restricted normal activities in adjustment to illness and disability: A model of depressed affect. *Rehabilitation Psychology, 43*, 327–347.

Wilson, D. S. (2016). Intentional culture change. *Current Opinion in Psychology, 8*, 190–193. https://doi.org/10.1016/j.copsyc.2015.12.012

Wilson, D. S., Hayes, S. C., Biglan, A., & Embry, D. D. (2014). Evolving the future: Toward a science of intentional change. *Behavioral and Brain Sciences, 37*(4), 395–416. https://doi.org/10.1017/S0140525X13001593

Wilson, E. G. (2008). *Against happiness: In praise of melancholy*. Farrar, Straus and Giroux.

Wilson, T. D. (2002). *Strangers to ourselves: Discovering the adaptive unconscious*. Harvard University Press.

Wilson, T. D. (2011). *Redirect: The surprising new science of psychological change*. Little, Brown & Co.

Wilson, T. D. (2022). What is social psychology? The construal principle. *Psychological Review, 129*(4), 873–889. https://doi.org/10.1037/rev0000373

Wilson, T. D., & Gilbert, D. T. (2003). Affective forecasting. In M. P. Zanna (Ed.), *Advances in experimental social psychology* (Vol. 35, pp. 345–411). Academic Press.

Wilson, T. D., Wheatley, T., Meyers, J. M., Gilbert, D. T., & Axsom, D. (2000). Focalism: A source of durability bias in affective forecasting. *Journal of Personality and Social Psychology, 78*, 821–836. https://doi.org/10.1037/0022-3514.78.5.821

World Health Organization. (2001). *International classification of functioning, disability, and health*. World Health Organization.

World Health Organization. (2013). *World report on disability*. World Health Organization. http://whqlibdoc.who.int/publications/2011/9789240685215_eng.pdf

World Health Organization (2023, March 23). Disability. https://www.who.int/news-room/fact-sheets/detail/disability-and-health

Wright, B. A. (Ed.). (1959). *Psychology and rehabilitation*. American Psychological Association. https://doi.org/10.1037/10539-000

Wright, B. A. (1960). *Physical disability: A psychological approach*. Harper & Row. https://doi.org/10.1037/10038-000

Wright, B. A. (1964). Spread in adjustment to disability. *Bulletin of the Menninger Clinic, 28*(4), 198–208.

Wright, B. A. (1972). Value-laden beliefs and principles for rehabilitation psychology. *Rehabilitation Psychology, 19*(1), 38–45. https://doi.org/10.1037/h0090869

Wright, B. A. (1975). Sensitizing outsiders to the position of the insider. *Rehabilitation Psychology, 22*, 129–135. https://doi.org/10.1037/h0090869

Wright, B. A. (1983). *Physical disability: A psychosocial approach* (2nd ed.). Harper & Row. https://doi.org/10.1037/10589-000

Wright, B. A. (1987). Human dignity and professional self-monitoring. *Journal of Applied Rehabilitation Counseling, 18*(4), 12–14. https://doi.org/10.1891/0047-2220.18.4.12

Wright, B. A. (1988). Attitudes and the fundamental negative bias. In H. E. Yuker (Ed.), *Attitudes towards persons with disabilities* (pp. 3–21). Springer.

Wright, B. A. (1989). Extension of Heider's ideas to rehabilitation psychology. *American Psychologist, 44*, 525–528. https://doi.org/10.1037/0003-066X.44.3.525

Wright, B. A. (1991). Labeling: The need for greater person-environment individuation. In C. R. Snyder & D. R. Forsyth (Eds.), *Handbook of social and clinical psychology: The health perspective* (pp. 469–487). Pergamon Press.

Wright, B. A. (1993). Division of Rehabilitation Psychology: Roots, guiding principles, and a persistent concern. *Rehabilitation Psychology, 38*(1), 63–65. https://doi.org/10.1037/h0085242

Wright, B. A., & Lopez, S. J. (2009). Widening the diagnostic focus: A case for including human strengths and environmental resources. In C. R. Snyder & S. J. Lopez (Eds.), *Handbook of positive psychology* (2nd ed., pp. 71–88). Oxford University Press. https://doi.org/10.1093/oxfordhb/9780195187243.013.0008

Wu, J., & Fiske, S. T. (2019). Disability's incompetence-but-warm stereotype guides selective empathy: Distinctive cognitive, emotional, and neural signatures. In D. S. Dunn (Ed.), *Understanding the experience of disability: Perspectives from social and rehabilitation psychology* (pp. 39–51). Oxford University Press.

Young, S. (2012, July 3). "We're not here for your inspiration." *The Drum*. http://www.abc.net.au/news/2012-07-03/young-inspiration-porn/4107006

Yuker, H. E. (Ed.). (1988). *Attitudes towards persons with disabilities*. Springer.

Yuker, H. E. (1994). Variables that influence attitudes toward people with disabilities: Conclusions from the data. *Journal of Social Behavior and Personality, 9*, 3–22.

Zapata, M. A. (2020). Disability affirmation and acceptance predict hope among adults with physical disabilities. *Rehabilitation Psychology, 65*(3), 291–298. https://doi.org/10.1037/rep0000364

Zupan, M. (2006). *Gimp: When life deals you a crappy hand, you can fold—or you can play it*. HarperCollins.

Index

For the benefit of digital users, indexed terms that span two pages (e.g., 52–53) may, on occasion, appear on only one of those pages.

Tables and figures are indicated by an italic *t* and *f* following the page number.